SO-ARJ-359

Shades of Love and Loss

CARING FOR A **PARTNER** WITH **DEMENTIA**

Dr. Nina Krebs

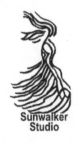

Sunwalker
Studio

Sunwalker Studio
1250 Newell Ave. Ste. I #147
Walnut Creek CA 94596
www.ninabkrebs.com

For further information go to www.ninabkrebs.com

All rights reserved. No part of this book may be reproduced or transmitted in any form or by any means, electronic or mechanical, including photocopying, recording, or any information storage and retrieval system, without permission in writing from the publisher.

This is a work of creative nonfiction. Family names are used with permission.

Disclaimer: SHADES OF LOVE AND LOSS provides help for partners and caregivers, but this book is not a substitute for professional, legal or financial advice. Every situation is different.

Book design and cover by Rudy Ramos
Author photo by Slavic Paleny
Illustrations are by the author

2019 © Dr. Nina Krebs

ISBN: 978-1-7332612-0-3 (trade paper)
ISBN: ISBN: 978-1-7332612-1-0 (ebook)
Printed in the United States of America

*Of course this book is dedicated to
Dave Krebs
and our family.
And to the millions of patients, families and caregivers
whose daily lives
are clamped
in dementia's relentless embrace.*

Table of Contents

Dear Reader,

Thank you for taking time to read my book. If you are interested in this topic you are probably caring for someone with dementia or know someone who is. I've written the book from the point of view of caring for my husband, Dave. Even though the content may apply to other relationships, I'm using the word *partner* to describe my loved one. I hope my thoughts and experience will be helpful, and you will feel less alone in this sad, challenging journey. As I share my caregiver experience, here's what I hope will be useful for you:

1. *The beginning of dementia is subtle and not likely to be recognized for what it is.* Like Carl Sandburg's "Fog," dementia comes creeping in on little cat feet and then sits on silent haunches looking around. Unlike the fog, which moves on, dementia stays and becomes more pronounced. As your partner becomes more anxious and rigid with increased memory failures and impaired ability to track, you may feel that they are choosing to be this way and become impatient and angry, even feel betrayed.

2. *Self-doubt enters, along with agitation, anger and impatience.* Shame at having these feelings is likely to be part of the mix. You find yourself acting like someone you wouldn't recognize. Family members or friends might point out your hostility and ask you about it. They may be critical of you. All of this is part of the process and does not mean that you are a bad person. They do not see what is happening in your life on a daily basis. It might help to ask them to come stay with your loved one while you take a little vacation.

3. *The medical establishment may not be aware or helpful in providing you with information about the early stages of dementia.* This leaves you in a vacuum feeling like you must be missing something or doing something wrong. In fact, you may have all kinds of feelings you haven't had before and not recognize what they are about. It is difficult to suggest to your loved one that an evaluation of his or her

mental state would be helpful, even after you begin to understand what is happening.

4. *You may feel disloyal or as though you're being unfairly critical when you begin noticing something is wrong with your partner.* When you start checking with friends about whether they have noticed anything, you are likely to discover that they have seen changes but didn't want to say anything.

5. *One of the first things you can do for yourself is work at clarifying your feelings.* Feel them. Listen to them. Label them. Write about them or make art about them. Understand that you have real reasons for feeling the way that you do. When you are clear about what you are feeling and why, you can address the related issues and problem solve.

6. *As you become clearer, hopefully, you will be motivated to get help in finding out what is going on, i.e. a neurological evaluation for your loved one.* This is difficult because it means acknowledging that something is wrong and asking your partner to cooperate in getting more information. You can no longer deny that your life is changing, and you can't stop it. If you can't figure it out for yourself – and most people can't – get help from family, friends and/or professionals (a therapist) about how to talk with your loved one about what you are observing. It helps to have good examples of impaired behavior that are recognizable to that person. "We need help…" might be a way to begin the conversation.

7. *You will need help. No one can care for a partner with dementia alone.* Whatever your feelings are about asking for help, now is the time to become good at it. I found this step incredibly difficult because I didn't know whom to ask. I had moved from the city where I had lived for decades to a dense urban area where I had no social network and didn't know the territory. I had no clue about resources for elders or people with dementia, or for someone in my situation. Nor was I prepared for the financial shock that was in store for me. Your partner needs care, but it need not, and cannot, be provided solely by you. Find someone you like who is in similar straits and create a buddy system for doing what you need to do.

8. *As dementia claims more and more of your partner, your responsibilities grow exponentially.* Decision-making becomes your job and includes major life decisions, which you probably made jointly before. You become responsible for another person's wellbeing and everything that it involves. You can no longer rely on your partner for consultation on important issues, so it is essential to *find trusted resources with whom you can consult*: financial advisor, friends, professionals who work with elders. You also become responsible for all the logistics that keep your household together.

9. *Strategies for dealing with your partner's resistance to change may require you to abandon authenticity in communication in order to accomplish goals for care.* I found it necessary to manipulate, lie, sneak and act dumb, after years of having a relationship based on open communication. You are unlikely to be able to jointly make decisions about moving, taking over finances, doing all the driving, getting help, or making legal decisions, among other necessities of life.

10. *Your aging process is happening concurrently with the deepening of your partner's dementia.* You are faced with the necessity of making decisions about the end of your partner's life as well as your own. Legal, financial and spiritual arrangements all need attention.

I have listed ten items that catalogue issues someone caring for a partner with dementia is likely to face. There are undoubtedly more I haven't included. Item #11, which deals with self-care, counter-balances the other ten. Mindfully taking care of yourself is the bedrock upon which the structure of your well-being rests.

11. *Learn how to take care of yourself in at least two modes: self-maintenance and self-nourishment. Commit to your self-care program.* The basis of the partnership – emotional support, sharing the workload and finances, joint pleasures, fun vacations and holidays, romance and intimacy – are going, or are gone forever. How do you rebuild your life? You will provide most of your own care, and that requires time, energy, money and discipline. Identify and create what will work for you to reduce stress and support your energy. It isn't a luxury to take

care of yourself; it's a necessity. People get sick and die in the role of caregiver from lack of self-care. Just as it is necessary to clarify your feelings, it is essential to figure out what you need and find ways to provide for yourself. I spend nearly three hours daily engaged in my routine: a two-mile walk, Qigong practice (meditation) and music practice. You can find help and support, and it is important to do so, but only you can create and maintain the container for your self-care. No one else can do this for you.

You are not alone. You only need to mention to someone that you are a caregiver for a person with dementia, and a story will come from the other about a family member or friend in the same situation.

Love and best wishes on your journey,
Nina Krebs

Prologue

Live and love every moment you have with the person
who is your soul mate.
Seeing that person slip into no person's land is surreal.
Frog in the water.
A little thing here.
A little thing there.
And soon it takes six interactions to explain the next step.
A blank look.

Nina Krebs
January 2015

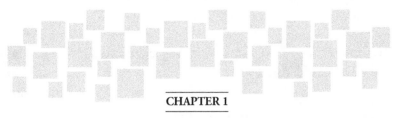

CHAPTER 1

Introduction

I belong to a network nobody wants to join, but our membership is growing fast. If you're in the net, we probably share daily experiences with our life partners that are uncomfortable, to say the least. In fact, some of us diminish or hide the realities of everyday life from family and friends. And from ourselves.

Dementia, including Alzheimer's, isn't contagious in the same way the flu is. Its collateral damage is psychological, but it can turn perniciously physical as well. The shift from *partner* to *caregiver* demands a new stance with your spouse or life partner and with yourself. The unwelcome journey from limbo to conscious caregiving has obscure causes and subtle impact like none other. It affected my husband directly while ricocheting with deadening force into me.

For the purpose of this book, I will use the term dementia as a generic descriptor. Briefly, this syndrome is associated with aging, and the symptoms are pronounced enough to interfere with an individual's ability to carry on daily life. Memory loss, impairment of the ability to track time, place and events, confusion, and bad judgment are present in varying degrees. As the patient's brain changes, physical impairments occur also, such as notable changes in gait and posture, as well as issues with balance. Behavior may become socially inappropriate, without the patient's awareness that anything is wrong.

There are many kinds of dementia, the most common of which is Alzheimer's Syndrome. Statistics range widely, but roughly 60 to 80 percent of people with dementia have Alzheimer's, although this condition can't be formally diagnosed until there is an autopsy. Diagnosis and definition of dementia is complex, controversial, and not the subject of this book.

The focus here is on caregiving. For many of us, taking care of a partner may be added to other family caregiving tasks. Among other life responsibilities, how do you take care of your partner when managing his or her own care is no longer possible? Where does caring for yourself reside under those conditions? What is the difference between caring for someone and caregiving?

Taking care of your partner who has dementia changes your life, whether you provide care at home, have help at home, or arrange for your partner to live elsewhere. The shift may be gradual, but ultimately you alter the way you spend your time, your energy, and your money. Your circle of friends is likely to vary, and you may find yourself moving, even though you never intended to do so.

As a partner in this process, we lose our easy life rhythm in the haven we co-created. The ways we know and understand ourselves in relationship shrink. We no longer have time and energy for our own interests. The inextricably melded dynamic of self-loss through caregiving determines daily choices. Adult children and grandchildren in families where one person is a caregiver for a partner suffer the loss of both. The caregiver's energy is likely to flow to the partner's care rather than to the family in general.

If you are caring for your life partner with dementia, I wrote this book for you, as well as for me. My goal is to help our network appreciate how much we have in common as we bear the loneliness and grief of caring for a partner with Alzheimer's or one of the other dementias. Much of the content applies to anyone who is a caregiver for a person with dementia, or even other disabilities, but the world I know is that of the spouse caregiver. The profound loss of a life partner to dementia includes the disappearance of a large chunk of one's own being that is unique to the spouse or life-partner relationship.

How do two seniors, one of whom has dementia, embrace the aging process and continue living the values that guided their lives and their long careers (in our case) in mental health? These values for me included unconditional positive regard, compassion, direct communication, effective conflict management and personal responsibility. Does my background in psychology help or hurt? What does it bring to every day at life's end? How do we embrace the new normal? These were questions I asked myself.

In today's frenetic world, caring for a disabled elder partner falls squarely on the other aged partner's shoulders. If there are adult children, they are likely to be consumed by jobs and their own families, and may live in a different town or state. Some public or institutional resources may be available, but finding them is like taking on a whole new career. The expense of professional help is overwhelming, if not out of reach, for most families. When churches or other organizations help, they certainly provide a boost, but they do not cover the bulk of time or needs.

Spouse or life-partner caregivers comprise a small portion of people who care for relatives at home. Around twelve per cent of those caring for disabled family members care for spouses. Most family caregivers are serving other relatives, not their life partners and soul mates. (Russo, Francine. "The Givers," *Scientific American Mind,* November/December 2016, pp.28-35.)* It makes sense that the percentage of spouse caregivers is relatively low just because spouses tend to be as advanced in age as the person with the diagnosis. (*You will find more information about * items in the* REFERENCES *section at the back of the book.*)

Caregivers, especially spouses and life partners, find ourselves overwhelmed with responsibility we don't want and flooded with feelings we can't name. The beginning for any of the dementias is usually subtle and not likely to be recognized for what it is. The caregiver is often deeply into the process of abandoning her or his way of life without consciously acknowledging that the relationship is dissolving and rearranging itself.

When I first began noticing my husband Dave's changing behavior, I attributed it to the aging process in general. His seniority of seven years didn't make much difference at the beginning of our relationship, but as time passed he became increasingly anxious and less emotionally available. I had no idea that these indicators were symptoms of a degenerative disease, so I adjusted as needed and went on with life. Now I know I was seeing the early signs of Alzheimer's and that our lives were about to change in ways I never would have predicted.

We were well past the initial diagnosis and into the progress of the disease before I decided to write this book. Even after I was clear about what was happening and had the benefit of having kept a journal for years, I pushed aside the idea of sharing my bumbling agony in any public way. Going through it was hard enough. Who needed to revisit the journey with the specificity required to tell the story so it might be meaningful to others? The possibility nagged me for at least two years. Finally, in an effort to focus and clarify my own thoughts and feelings, I decided to dive in and write.

When I actually started writing and talked with a few people about the book, one friend said, "I never read these books about a caregiver's experience, because they're usually just that person's catharsis." Good point. On the other hand, I recently met a woman whose mid-stage Alzheimer's-diagnosed spouse was abusing her psychologically and chasing her around the house. Because he was her partner, she saw it as her job to stay in the house with him. It hadn't occurred to her to seek an alternative, though she's a brilliant woman with financial resources, perfectly capable of devising a solution to her nightmare. We lose our powers of observation and good judgment right along with our partners when we are *in* the situation. Because of this loss of insight, I concluded that painful as it may be to write or read, a book describing my experience could be useful.

Wrapped in self-doubt, I wanted to ignore my ugly thoughts and feelings because they didn't fit my self-image. I hated the way I felt and tried not to acknowledge my agitated depression, hostile feelings, and escapist fantasies. The book is my attempt to portray those emotions in their indistinct but unremitting shades and claim them, despite their unacceptability to others or to me. I have included intimate self-disclosures, behavioral descriptions, and professional insights to create what I hope is a multi-dimensional view of the slow shift in my husband's personality, our partnership, our family, and my path alongside him from partner to caregiver. You may recognize parts of yourself and your experience in these pages.

If there is a way through the dementia caregiver morass, it is necessary to be clear about what hurts, to embrace the pain, to know that the anguish is real, and to find ways to face life's truth and deal with it. The last segment is the hardest because the ways to move into a better place may involve making choices and decisions you would never have predicted or believed within your capacity.

My hope is that knowing you are not alone will offer solace as you read. We all age differently, and people with dementia may share similarities, but each is unique and affected differently by changes in the brain. The same is true for partner caregivers. What helps one person may seem terrible to another. I'll be describing the path my family and

I took in caring for Dave with no implication that this is the "right" way to proceed. People in other cultures, religions or social groups have different values and ways of working with a spouse or family member who has failing health with dementia.

No matter what the approach, my emphasis is on creating time and opportunity for the caregiver to care for herself or himself. Support from family, friends and professional helpers and willingness to request and accept that help is central. When I began to understand, not just "know," the importance of self-care and take it seriously, I began to trust that I would manage my life again.

Only one person is qualified for your self-care job.

That person is you.

CHAPTER 2

Meet the
Author

The path leading to my chosen career as a therapist was oblique, emerging from what now seems like the Dark Ages. I grew up on the high desert in the little town of Winslow, Arizona. My parents owned a business there. I lived with them and my sister, Judy, in the same house on Elm Street from the time I was born until I graduated from high school and left for college at Arizona State (then) College.

As far as I could tell in 1956, when I graduated from high school, career choices for women were limited to being a nurse, a secretary, or a teacher. I chose teacher. After the first semester of my freshman year at college, I rarely returned to Winslow.

I married my college sweetheart following graduation. That fall I began my career as a high school English teacher in Tempe, Arizona. In 1962, we moved to my husband's home state of Indiana and had two daughters, Erica and Karen, who are now aged fifty plus. I had a seemingly perfect life in many ways, but I became deeply unhappy in the marriage and attempted to make things better by continuing my education. We moved from the farm where we lived in east central Indiana to a beautiful new home in the nearby town of Muncie so I could continue graduate work at Ball State University. My husband was a good person, but our choices at age 21 weren't valid for a lifetime. I was less and less able to pretend that life was okay through sheer will.

Like most middle class white women of my generation, I had been programmed from childhood to see myself as a wife and mother. A job or career could be part of my life, but not the main part. Education and the women's movement opened my eyes to other possibilities. I remember a moment while I was still living on the farm that my perspective changed in a big way. It was early morning. Feeling burdened by housework and toddler care, I was ironing my husband's twill work uniform in the playroom I had created in one of the farmhouse bedrooms. Watching *The Today Show* in the very early morning, I viewed Barbara Walters intelligently commenting on current events. "Why is she there, and I am here?" rocketed through my mind. I had been reading Betty Freidan's, *The Feminine Mystique,* * as well.

Clever though my plan was to enrich my life through more education, and as generous as my husband had been in making the move to Muncie for me, the hoped-for solution failed. I couldn't coerce myself into contentment or even a good level of getting by. Our divorce was final at the end of 1969. This emotional earthquake, known to family and ex-friends in Indiana as "that terrible divorce," continues to shed fallout. It wasn't an easy decision. I was on my own in a graduate program with two small children and what swelled into an 80-hour workweek.

My antidote to the stress was to fall in love with a cowboy, a fellow doctoral student, who was philosophically opposed to commitment in a relationship. It was the late '60s, and I was into liberation. I thought. I had spent 1967, "The Summer of Love," on a Midwest farm, remodeling a 100-year-old farmhouse while mothering toddlers. I reveled in my new life: mostly interesting classes, new friends, an internship, and an exhilarating relationship. The latter was a challenging Kawasaki ride that metaphorically crashed and burned, making me a sad but wiser woman.

The non-academic part of my education was as important to my understanding of life as the work for which I received a diploma was. Stepping beyond my conventional upbringing fueled my capacity to make choices that were aligned with my perceived wants and needs and to deal with negative consequences if they occurred. I began to trust myself in a whole new way and rely less on the judgments of others. I could suffer loss, recover, and gain new strength in the process.

The girls and I survived graduate school and, I found a job as a psychologist in the Counseling Center at California State University, Sacramento, where I stayed for five years.

By the time I finished my doctorate, found a job, and moved to California, it was OK with me that a loving, committed relationship would be absent from my life. Fine. I had two beautiful daughters whom

I loved like crazy, the capacity to support myself, and who needed a man? I certainly didn't need or want someone to "take care of me," as if that were the way it worked. I wouldn't trade my hard-earned self-determination for romance, companionship, and a security that wasn't secure at all.

No one was more surprised than I was when I met Dave, and my story shifted.

In a very short time, we stepped into an equal partnership where things worked, or if they didn't, we stayed with the process until we figured it out. We had our parallel professional lives, in which I could be as independent as I needed or wanted to be, and our joint family life with its aura of comfort and security. The girls matured and went their ways. We enjoyed an active social life and the freedom to travel on long weekends as well as during the customary August break psychotherapists took back then.

Dave and I could carry on our independent lives within the relationship so I had adequate mobility and enough space for my own projects and interests to feel nourished and fulfilled. I adored Dave and treasured spending time with him, but I didn't depend on him to keep me interested and happy. We cooked, hiked, joked, made a king-size quilt together, relished time with family and friends, travel and art, and we created a rich relationship. Life was good. We married in 1973.

After five years at the counseling center, I got the itch to be outside the university setting and moved into private practice downtown with group of four other psychologists, including Dave. We created a center for providing psychological services to individuals, families and organizations.

Dave and I had a wonderful time with our colleagues building and succeeding in our new business. We defied the prediction made by a university colleague that we would fail within the year and wish we were back in the fold. The format for our psychology practice changed over the years, but Dave and I maintained our parallel practices until he retired in 1994.

When I retired in 1998, my main focus had been family and work. I managed to write some books along the way* and varied my work life by doing both clinical and organizational practice. The latter was done in partnership with my brilliant, creative, irreverent friend, Mary Bolton. Our common interests in women's issues propelled us on a challenging and rewarding journey through the consulting world.

Like other second-wave feminists, I was determined to do it all, and so I gave work and family life my best effort. Music had been a major anchor during childhood and adolescence, but I abandoned that pursuit for forty years, partly due to lack of time, partly because I wouldn't give myself permission to indulge. With work and family, I had little time to devote to the arts. When I closed my psychology practice, I happily approached the world of making and appreciating visual art and reconnected with myself by playing music.

At one point I had considered majoring in music but had abandoned that idea. At the time, I didn't realize I was leaving behind a significant part of myself. I wasn't an outstanding musician, nor did I have the dedication to become one. Nonetheless, listening to and playing music was my go-to place for enjoyment, self-nourishment, and stress reduction. It wasn't about performance. Making music is a visceral part of me. Much later in my life, reclaiming that part after its 40-year absence empowered and enlivened me.

My feminist view of marriage was that Dave and I each needed to be independent, responsible adults, equal partners, and to manage our individual lives, (including our own emotional health), while being connected and supportive in our relationship. To me this meant we helped each other, as needed, and shared our resources. We created a division of labor that worked for our family. We could rely on and trust each other to follow through with what we agreed on. I called this concept in marriage reciprocity, an equal and trustworthy give and take between a couple who face life together. Love and mutual respect made sharing easy and enjoyable.

While the girls grew up, Dave and I shared responsibility for their upbringing, although in major issues and decisions, we agreed that I had the last word because I was the biological parent. Dave was emotionally supportive and financially generous with Erica and Karen from the beginning of our relationship.

Despite my investment in my education and career, our family has always been my priority. Our daughters are both extraordinary people and have been from infancy. When I left my family home in Winslow, I really LEFT. I assumed that when Erica and Karen grew up, they would do the same, and I would see them only rarely. To my great joy, that has not been the case. They kept coming back to spend time with us, look in on our lives, hang out, and invite us into their space. I am touched and grateful for their love, loyalty, presence, and especially in these later years, for their ever-accessible help.

My sister Judy, another pillar in my life, and I had a major falling out after Mother's death in 1973, but thanks to a courageous intervention by her son, Nick, and her generous forgiveness, we are now true friends. I rely on her humor, talent, creativity, and support and offer her the same. We create opportunities for travel together that take me away from the caregiver life and provide fun and the nourishment of shared history and loving companionship.

We all have our baggage, and somehow life gives us the persistence to face repeated worn out challenges and failures, occasionally in recognizable form, but often not. It seemed to me, when I was growing up, that my mother was trapped in a relationship and lifestyle she couldn't escape. My parents' alcoholic routine was such that Mother did not have the independence and resources to leave, but staying was miserable. I determined to make sure that I could support myself financially and manage life on my own. Even after I had completed my doctorate, with two young daughters to support, fear of becoming a victim revisited me.

Years before I recognized Dave's distancing behavior as dementia, the connection between us began to come apart. I found myself explaining jokes. Dave asked about the recipe for lasagna – there had never been one – his stepdad had taught him to make it. I became increasingly responsible for both sides of the relationship and all its concerns.

The world began to tilt.

As Dave became increasingly impaired, I was less able to live the life I had known with him. Before the word Alzheimer's entered Dave's medical record my life slipped into the tedium of managing our daily requirements. In 2013, we moved from Sacramento where we had lived for four decades in order to be near Karen and her family in the San Francisco Bay Area and closer to Erica and her husband, Rex, in Santa Cruz. I no longer had my long-standing social network and casual acquaintances, nor did I have the time or the energy to take classes, write, or make art. My energy seeped away. Sharing, joy, and the give and take in our relationship evaporated.

Couples get to choose from an array of relationship styles about how to organize their lives, starting with a traditional model where the man is in charge and the woman serves him. Children in such families are expected to be seen but not heard. The household in which Judy and I grew up followed this plan. For sure I knew I didn't want to re-create that style. I had never understood why people were subservient because they were female.

When I was a child, Amelia Addington (Meme), a Native American woman of the Tohono O'odham tribe, lived with us and was like an emotional mother for Judy and me. She shared the ways of her culture with us, and we spent significant time with her and her (mainly) Hopi friends outside our home. We loved going to Hopi dances at the mesa pueblos north of Winslow and felt very much at home in that environment. Our mother said we didn't know we were "white" until we went to school. From Meme we learned that our middle-class life style was not the only way families were organized. People we knew and loved dealt with life and family concerns differently. Our worldview wasn't the only one. Meme's influence shaped many of my tastes and interests and remains a major part of my identity.

When Dave and I got together, we were both clear that we were partners with equal power and authority in our relationship. We shared financial responsibility proportional to our income. We made decisions together, and when we disagreed, we discussed the situation until a plan evolved. We relied on each other for help and support. We traveled together and shared other activities, but we also supported each other in our individual interests, trips and undertakings. When this model began to shatter I felt the walls closing in.

Growing up I was taught that I was responsible for what I could see. If my friend spilled the milk, I should wipe it up. If someone needed help getting across the street or directions, my job was to assist. Dishes left on the table were mine to pick up. Later in life this outlook translated to being friendly, helpful, and supportive to family members and other people without being asked. I was supposed to know what others needed and help them, which was the beginning of empathy training for me. Western hospitality was a tradition at home and in our little town. Not until I left Winslow and was in college did I seriously question these assumptions.

In early adulthood I learned that we deserve and need to have personal boundaries, that it's OK to say no to requests from others, and that I was responsible for myself but not for everyone around me. My training as a therapist and then years of practice in that profession provided layers of refinement about the subject of personal boundary management and who is responsible for what in a primary relationship, family, job site, or the world.

As Dave's personal competence slipped, responsibility loomed large in my vocabulary. His actions and decisions were increasingly erratic because dementia's failing memory and bad judgment resulted in poor choices about even the simplest things. Ultimately, how much responsibility was mine? And for what? And for how long?

Especially early in the development of Dave's illness, I was at war with myself because I couldn't absorb what was happening to him or to me in any meaningful way. When I could nab my emotional reactions, they weren't acceptable to me. Why was I ready to scream because Dave had asked three times which of the buckets - the word he began using for any container - was the right one for the plastic bottle he held in his hand, its remaining contents dribbling to the floor? This act seemed so small, considering that I'm not a fastidious housekeeper, and the disposal of one plastic bottle is not a matter of paramount importance.

I didn't recognize myself. I felt like a stranger who easily lost her patience in a fizz of agitation, not my usual style. In the early stages of dementia, much of a partner-caregiver's experience remains invisible to family members and friends. What family and friends see is someone who seems hostile and agitated for no apparent reason. For a long time our daughters who didn't see us at home frequently, missed the changes that were in progress. Dave stopped driving when we moved to the Bay Area, but since we still had a beautiful life style and could do pale versions of many of the things we had always done, like go out to dinner or to concerts and the theater, outward appearances weren't noticeably different.

What others weren't seeing was that life had become increasingly bland at home with sports on television providing a focus for Dave. Shared tasks, banter, easy give and take over dinner were gone. Getting through the day without collapsing into that old familiar sensation, depression, became a focus for me, although I didn't see it that way at the time. Dave was the center of the household, sitting in his recliner in our living room, dozing and flipping through channels on TV. I observed that he wasn't looking for anything specific to watch. He was just staring at the screen. And, I was watching him.

The discrepancy between surface normalcy and my inner experience compounded my confusion and loneliness. I didn't really get that my life had changed drastically, and much of what I had taken for granted for decades had disappeared. Poignantly, by 2013, I lived in the one part of the world where I had longed to be for much of my adult life, forty minutes by Bay Area Rapid Transit (BART) from the rich art world of San Francisco and the rest of the Bay Area. Sadly, though, my responsibilities at home made it not impossible, but very difficult to get there.

I was in exactly the position I had spent my life avoiding.

Trapped.

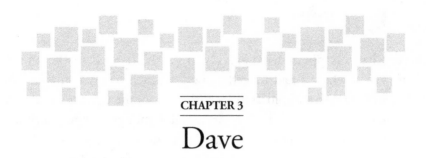

CHAPTER 3

Dave

Dave Krebs was 39 when I met him in my job search nearing the end of my work in graduate school. I had no idea what was in store for me! Dave was a psychologist at the university counseling center where I hoped to get a job. The selection process was set up so that I met individually with senior staff members for in-depth interviews, and had lunch with a small group. I was exhausted, having taken an expensive, quick break from my unrelenting schedule in graduate school to look for a job. Interviewing is nerve wracking, and I was on edge, working hard to appear competent, professional, and confident at the same time. The day was long. Dave's interview was last.

When it was his turn to talk with me, Dave invited me to his office and began the interview in a casual way. His handsome, urbane appearance caught me off guard, but his easy smile and relaxed body language made me feel welcome. Nearly fifty years later, I can visualize the scene and even remember what I was wearing, (and the fat run I discovered in the back of my stockings when I got home) though I can't recall the exact content of our conversation. What I'll never forget is the emotional quality of that meeting. Dave listened to me. This articulate, fine-looking guy heard what I said and respectfully took our conversation to the next level. He asked questions that encouraged me to explain my work and interests and then followed up so I felt he truly wanted to know who I was. I was instantly attracted to him and liked him. Unfortunately, he was married, so I was clear nothing would happen in the romance department.

I expected skilled listening and communication from a therapist. It took getting to know Dave, though, to understand that this wasn't just his counseling style. He was deeply interested in people and had a bottomless well of empathy, different in this way from any man I had known before.

I did get the job at the counseling center, and, to my delight, discovered that Dave and I shared professional and philosophical viewpoints and had much to talk about. Despite the fact that he was more experienced and held higher academic rank than I, he welcomed me as an equal, and that level platform never changed.

In late October of my first year on the staff, a colleague invited all of us to a party at his house. It was a lavishly simple affair featuring excellent wine, good food, and easy camaraderie. The open California-style home with its white carpets, swimming pool, and subtle lighting felt warm and welcoming. Toward the end of the evening, lingering with my new colleagues and talking with Dave, someone asked him about the houseboat trip he had taken the previous summer. His party smile dropped and his face saddened as he thought about his answer. "It was OK," he began, "but seven days on that boat helped me clarify my decision to get a divorce. I've been living alone since July."

"OH, NO!" I blurted. My blatant tone didn't communicate sympathy. I wanted to disappear as the loud words turned surprised glances my way. There was no way to cover my blaring non sequitur. Like Houdini, Dr. Krebs had slipped from the airtight compartment of married man in which my heart had chained him. Now, he stood smiling at me, asking if he could refill my drink.

He invited me to dinner the following evening. By the middle of the next month he moved in to the little apartment I had rented for the girls and me. No transition. It was as if we had been invented in different soul factories at the same moment, clanged together and stuck. I had never been happier. I adored Dave and loved being with him. Nothing about him, the way he treated me, or anything he did would make me think this relationship would dissolve any time soon, or maybe ever.

My attraction to Dave was super-charged. I fell in love with him over and over, and I wasn't disappointed. He responded in kind, making me feel valued and happy. It was hard to stay business-like in our professional setting, and from time to time our standards slipped. Years later an ex-client told me, she was offended when she saw him pat me on the backside when we were walking down the hall, and she let me know it was very unprofessional. Our rapid cohabitation wasn't unusual for the times, but it felt daring to me. It also felt just right. We began our life together and enjoyed our adventurous relationship.

Erica and Karen were included from the beginning in getting to know this new person who had landed in the center of their lives. This was not easy for them. Dave took all of us to Monterey for a weekend in an attempt to include the girls and have family time. We stayed in a beautiful hotel on the beach. At sunset we were out strolling on the sand by the turquoise water with its gold-brushed foam. "Look at the beautiful ocean!" I said to the girls. "I hate that ugly old ocean," Karen said, making it perfectly clear that she wanted nothing to do with the whole thing.

In the beginning, I saw this partnership, despite my dazzled state, as an experiment, not necessarily anything that would last forever. From day one, Dave was present and took care of business, including cooking, laundry and keeping the household together. He treated Erica and Karen as if they were his own children financially and emotionally, and helped them in any way he could. He won them over, and they love him deeply. As a distant relative shocked me by saying about him, "He didn't even molest them." That idea was so far from Dave's persona, the comment blew my mind and still does.

Over time, if I anticipated Dave would be angry or critical of me, that didn't occur. One of his favorite sayings was, "We're all more human than anything else." Another was, "I'm sure you (or whoever) didn't do that on purpose." He looked for the best in people and was habitually kind. He was good to me from the beginning.

His core capacity for empathy was one of the last of Dave's strengths to diminish, and the kindness remains. I have been dealing with the impaired Dave for so long, it is painful and probably impossible to recapture and describe the person I fell in love with, a man who became an enthusiastic, present, and immensely supportive partner for years. He was someone who knew how to be in a relationship in a consistent and loving way. I was fortunate to share many happy decades with Dave, and my gratitude for that time sustains me now.

It was 1971 when we met, and second wave, or post-structural feminism was in its early stages. Dave was not a chauvinist. From the time I met him, I sensed that he truly respected women in general and me as an equal, competent person. He was gentle and supportive in every possible way. The exceptions were short lived. Early in our relationship, he had a couple of temper outbursts, not toward me, but toward others. He was a big, strong guy, and the violence in these flare-ups scared me. I told him that kind of behavior was a deal breaker for me. It never happened again.

Dave knew how to be emotionally present in a clear, no nonsense way. I'm tempted to say he was innately emotionally supportive, but I'm not sure that is possible. From the beginning of our relationship, I was assertive about what I needed and wanted, a style very different from my early learning about being a woman. Each time I pushed a boundary, I would expect a negative response, but that didn't come. Sometimes we would problem-solve or negotiate, but he didn't imply that I was unreasonable or undeserving in any way. These strengths remained throughout our marriage.

When I met Dave, besides being gorgeous, he was physically active, in great shape, and loved sports. He took up jogging in the early 1970's, and ran nearly every day for years. When he could no longer run, he walked, either by himself or with me. He didn't participate in team sports after I knew him, but he loved watching football and basketball on TV and considered himself a jock. He still embraces that identity.

The part that is hardest to describe now is the fun and love between us. We were good partners. We enjoyed being together and undertook projects or trips that were engaging to do and then talk about afterward. We had long conversations about wide-ranging subjects over dinner with each other and with friends. We worked together and consulted with each other about professional issues of all kinds. We had different approaches to doing therapy (those differences widened) and yet, we understood each other's point of view and could help with that in mind.

Dave was responsible and reliable. He enjoyed life and would easily agree to going out for dinner, to a concert or some other adventure large or small. I dragged him to the symphony and art museums early in our relationship, and then he genuinely began enjoying this important part of my life. He participated actively when we traveled as a couple or with friends. He loved hiking and being outdoors and moved along a trail with athletic grace, even when he carried a pack. He resisted camping when I first proposed it, and then became a devotee.

We cajoled the girls into a camping trip early one winter, even though rain threatened. They resisted, wisely, but we went anyway. When it started to pour, they got to say, "See!! It's raining." Dave's reply was, "Ah, that's not rain. Those are fog stones," a joke that has lasted for years. When the kids' air mattresses floated in their tent and the Boy Scouts abandoned camp, we relented and headed for a motel.

Although he could be a worrier at times, Dave's general outlook on life was optimistic. He undertook a project like remodeling, moving into private practice, or planning a big trip with the expectation that the project would work out well. He was encouraging when the road got bumpy. This quality was one of the earliest affected by his aging and dementia. He became increasingly anxious, but it took me years to believe and adjust to the dissolution of his positive viewpoint.

Dave was highly qualified in the field of personality assessment and testified in court as an expert witness. As a therapist, he dealt with painful material or heated conflict in ways that people could hear and absorb From time to time I did co-therapy with him, and I admired his way with people who were in pain. His intuition bordered on psychic; his presence was calming without being overly solicitous.

Using his skill in assessment, Dave had served as a field selection officer for the Peace Corps on several occasions, traveling to Mexico, Brazil, and places in the United States before I knew him. From this experience, he developed an interest in learning Spanish and toward the end of his career began taking language classes at Sacramento City College. He attended an immersion program in San Luis Potosi, Mexico, and spent six weeks living with a family there, speaking only Spanish. He became fluent, read extensively in the language, and spoke Spanish with anyone he thought might respond in kind. After dementia took over, I heard him telling someone he had served in the Peace Corps in Tibet. What a surprise! Dave hadn't travelled in that part of the world.

Several years before he retired, Dave completed a post-doctorate degree in psychoanalysis, of which he was very proud. He modified his theoretical view significantly. His departure from our shared views of working with people meant that we rarely consulted with each other. This was a huge loss to me, a big shift from the early years of our time together. When he began talking seriously about retirement, it seemed that the time was right to take that step, and I supported him in his choice. His life-changing decision was in line with his long-held personal goals, creating a graceful close to his career.

I trusted I could carry the practice.

In 1994, upon his retirement, Dave had his social security and the savings we had accrued, thanks to the advice of our astute financial planner. The responsibility for producing income became mine. I needed to make $100,000 a year to keep the boat afloat, and I was doing it. Dave seemed content with his retirement decision, and it was OK with me. In a way, it was a relief that he was no longer in the practice. After he left the office, I realized I had been shepherding his schedule and acting as his office assistant.

Even in the early days of our relationship, Dave rarely reached out to make new friends, but he thoroughly enjoyed the people who frequented our business and social life, especially two local couples with whom we spent significant time. For reasons of their own, the men in these couples dropped out of our lives, creating a vacuum that never refilled. By the time these losses occurred, Dave had turned a corner, and I hadn't seen him go. I hadn't realized he no longer had the capacity to reach out for new friendships.

Just in case you're thinking, "Did this guy walk on water?" he didn't. He could be rigid and self-centered. At times, he would pontificate, give little psych theory lectures to our friends and me, despite the fact that we, too, were mental health professionals and had ideas and theories worth discussing. When he was right he was right! When confronted with something he didn't want to share, he would slide off the subject and psychologically disappear. He enhanced the truth from time to time, inflating his history or performance.

While Dave and I were partners in many ways, we had not started the offspring project together. We had some real differences in the area of child rearing: he thought I was too lenient, and I thought he was too strict. We mostly maintained our equilibrium, but at times I had recurring images of powerful horses tied to each of my limbs, running full tilt in all four directions. I felt caught between Dave and the girls who had conflicting needs and interests as well as different requirements for my time and attention. When conflict flared, I felt that rather than using his expertise to help us through a rough patch, Dave acted like another kid.

These family conflicts tore me up. Some days, sheer survival was all I could manage. I felt hypocritical working as a psychologist, doing family therapy, while having serious struggles at home. As long as I was around to dance to each family member's tune and orchestrate the discordant combo, we could manage some semblance of rhythm. The conflict burst out of control when I wasn't there to monitor. For sure I had my own flaws and wasn't always the consummate parent and partner. Having come from a patriarchal family where Mother propped up Daddy's ego rather than confronting him, I wasn't good in these complex situations. Although I was assertive about my own interests and needs, I avoided conflict among family members rather than taking it on. At the worst of the mess, we did seek help from a family therapist and were able to move on.

Like my sister Judy and I, Erica and Karen have diverse personalities. They will always have distinct points of view on many topics. From time to time, old differences surface and my need to control rears its frazzled head. With Dave's illness, stresses have softened. Our whole family has shown up, focused on doing what we need to do to support each other in the best possible ways.

Dave and I persevered and stumbled through parenthood and middle age, hand in hand, not always agreeing, but consistently able to sort jumbled emotions or crossed motives. We walked into another level of partnership, far beyond the lure of our early romance. I remain awed by Dave's loyalty and devotion, his willingness to meet the challenges of a blended family. I know I've contributed my part, but his tenacity and commitment wove a safety net that, for the most part, prevented slips and slides from becoming disasters.

The girls matured, and home life became simpler. We were involved in our various pursuits and doing well enough with them. I started seeing a therapist who helped me with many things, among them my unrealistic expectations for our family and myself. I learned to be less self-critical and began to relax more.

Relationship dynamics are never one-sided. Dave and I had our issues over time, some of which were never resolved. Having been a survivor and a risk taker to a certain degree, I assumed Dave also had those qualities. After all, I saw him as a big, strong guy with a Ph.D. who had a well-established career. He too was a survivor, but his life experiences had made it difficult for him to accept risk. When we took on a business venture, and it brinked on failure, his blood pressure soared, and all he wanted was out of it. I realized I had miscalculated.

Before dementia symptoms were obvious to me, Dave owned up to some ways he had exaggerated his accomplishments before I knew him. I didn't care about the content, but I felt betrayed and stupid that I hadn't confronted him when some of his stories didn't match my observations of his behavior. Whether it was denial on my part or intuition about Dave's impending condition, I didn't have the wherewithal to pursue the matter and express my disappointment and anger. I didn't think anything would be gained by doing so. I accepted his apology and moved forward.

Knowing someone well and intimately for years and weathering life's storms with them creates coatings of care that soften what would otherwise be logical responses to conflict. No relationship is perpetually smooth, and ours was wonderful in many ways, but there were bumps along the way. I think some form of disillusionment is likely in any long-term relationship at least once, and the wounds carry forward.

How we survive and integrate all this impacts our capacity to continue and cope with relationship and life endings. I can't help but think that some of my stowed resentment about the period in our life when Dave acknowledged his self-inflation fueled my anger before I knew his changing behavior was illness, not self-centeredness. It's one thing to deal with life if each person can haul his or her load and can work through differences and misunderstandings. The story gets scrambled when the bulk of the load shifts and neither party comprehends the turn.

From my perspective, Dave avoided exposing his own fears and defenses through therapy, and I was deeply frustrated and disappointed by that. What I perceived as his unwillingness to dismantle his narcissistic defenses* contributed to the way I slid into my old family pattern and sheltered his vulnerability rather than confronting him. And then dementia struck. We had a lot going for us and enjoyed many wonderful years. The evaporation of the magic between the two of us demoralized me.

I remember reading that Bruno Bettelheim*, one of my therapist heroes, had succumbed to Alzheimer's. I grieved to hear that this brilliant person who had contributed extensively to the field and the world had lost his mind and was no longer able to care for himself. And now I saw the same state in Dave, my magnificent, loving husband.

Layered shades of love and loss drift through us. Though I was married, I had lost the vitality of our relationship and the safety net of my partner's support.

I had become responsible for Dave's welfare in addition to my own.

CHAPTER 4

Diagnosis

When Dave turned 65, he subtly collapsed into old. Was that my projection? Was that when Alzheimer's symptoms began to surface? I remember thinking he seemed old, not all of a sudden, but markedly different. His gait shifted, and more rigidity and physical fragility were evident. Anxiety appeared at the smallest invitation. I was still working, and without being particularly conscious, I picked up more and more responsibility for daily living. I had my hands full.

Coinciding with his retirement in 1994, I noticed that Dave's essence, his vibrant energy field, had imperceptibly begun to shrink from gently strong and intelligent to anxious, flat, and tedious. Although it took me a long time to understand what was happening, the plaque and tangles* invading his brain were robbing him, and me, of his beautiful, complex mind while he was still walking among us. That incremental loss, like specks of stone washed away by decades of drips, blurs my memory of our many good years.

Additionally, there was Dave's preoccupation with his physical health. This had begun just a few years into our relationship, and it was symbolized for me by the blood pressure "cup" on the table by his chair in the family room. The proper term for that item is cuff, but I never questioned Dave's word for it. Why not? At first, he would take his blood pressure once or twice a day, and not necessarily every day. He would lie back in his recliner, mouth open like a gaping fish, relax, and then press the button on the BP gizmo. I thought he might wear the skin off his arm. When I entered a room after he began to take his BP, I would wait to say whatever I had to say, or leave. As time passed, he began measuring his blood pressure multiple times a day, and he wanted to read the numbers to me.

I asked him what his concern was, and he replied that taking his blood pressure was just a form of biofeedback. It helped him relax. This didn't make much sense to me, but I didn't probe. He would take it the first time, breathe deeply to relax some more, and repeat the process at least once, sometimes more. He denied that he was worried about anything in particular.

I was relieved if we took a little trip and he left the "cup" at home. It had become a fixture in our lives and another block in our communication. When Dave was fixated on taking his blood pressure, he was oblivious to anything else that might be going on around him.

Hindsight is 20:20. I can see now that some of Dave's behaviors that irritated and annoyed me, especially the anxiety that is an early hallmark for Alzheimer's, signaled the onset of the disease rather than coming from any choice on his part. His brain dysfunction was blocking flexibility and responsiveness, rendering him unable to deal with anything that landed outside his routine or expectations. I was seeing him as neurotic, anxious about some undefined concern that he wouldn't, or couldn't address directly. He was probably terrified.

If I were reading this, I would ask, "Why didn't you DO something?" Good question. I was trying, but not effectively. I saw the anxiety, but Dave wouldn't go to therapy, and I had no idea what else I could do to help. At the time I knew little about dementia of any kind and had no way to evaluate these behaviors as typical signs of that process. I was not seeing his anxiety as related to any physical condition, so I was trying to solve the wrong problem.

In addition to my ignorance, part of this quandary was my denial, another convoluted path. I didn't want to see what was happening. Explaining denial is impossible because when a person is in denial, they don't know it. When the veil lifts, everything seems obvious, and it is shocking to comprehend and acknowledge the obvious information that was unseen. I can see all those early signs now. I completely misdiagnosed them then.

When I look back on that time, it is difficult for me to believe what I wasn't seeing. Dave's affect and behavior were changing. The increments were tiny exaggerations of weird: a startle reaction without much stimulus, over concern about my safety or health, hyper vigilance while I was driving, stiff gestures with his hands, repetitive questions. No single one of these seemed serious or meaningful to me. I had no framework for understanding them other than thinking this is the way Dave was aging – withdrawing, becoming more needy and rigid, and worrying more.

His social behavior changed, too. In the past, Dave's way of being at a party or in a group was to find someone to talk with and spend significant time with that person and then move on to visit with someone else. He began clinging to me. When we attended friends' parties, art openings or other gatherings, I noticed that if I were talking with someone, Dave would stand near me, often slightly between the other person and me. I would shift my stance to regain contact and continue a conversation. I'm not much good at small talk or casual conversation, so social events became less interesting to me with this added layer of required attention. I found myself saying no thanks to invitations and recycling announcements of events I would usually have attended. I was withdrawing, too.

During the spring and summer of 2013, three major developments were in progress for Dave and me: more information about Dave's heart condition, his dementia diagnosis by a neurologist, and the decision to move from Sacramento to the Bay Area. These life-changing situations evolved concurrently in ways that were interwoven and confusing.

A cardiologist had seen Dave at least twice a year after it was discovered he had a heart murmur in the late 1980's. His diagnosis, aortic stenosis,* calcification of one of the valves that controls the flow of blood in the heart, had been confirmed. As early as the mid 1990's, knowing that blood flow and brain function were related, I explained some of Dave's behavior to the heart specialist. He said Dave might have some mild vascular dementia, nothing to worry about, part of the normal aging pattern. The doctor's informal assessment fit my observations and guesses, making it easier to dampen my initiative for scheduling a neurological evaluation. I was in the neverneverland between needing more information and supporting Dave's self esteem. I continued to live in this bind until I clearly understood that Dave's cognitive and behavioral symptoms indicated more than normal aging.

The aortic stenosis had progressed to the "severe" classification. Dave was not experiencing observable symptoms, but doctors with stethoscopes shook their heads when they listened. When he didn't feel well, my first job was to determine whether the issue was heart-related or something else. I used to be qualified to diagnose a variety of mental disorders but knew very little about cardiac malfunction. This lack of knowledge contributed to my anxiety and vigilance.

Dave's dementia was increasingly apparent to me, although I had yet to label it as such. I wasn't getting recommendations or confirmation from the medical establishment. Not one of Dave's physicians was saying, "Look, we need to assess what's happening with this guy's brain." They focused on his heart. I could have been more assertive about pushing for a diagnosis. I knew something was off, but I couldn't believe it enough to act. My usual consultant at a time like this would be Dave. *What do you think we should do?* I couldn't imagine how to bring this up to him.

Further, this dynamic was complicated by Dave's staunch unwillingness to subject himself to evaluation or treatment by members of his own profession, i.e. neuropsychologists or psychiatrists. It would have been a major fight, and I went along because I didn't think there was much to be gained. This was a big mistake. If I had known what we were facing, I could have become better informed and would have been more equipped to give myself permission to seek help. I thought if his condition was, indeed, some form of dementia, there was not much that could be done about it. I didn't understand it was going to be up to me to take over. Something could have been done for me.

Early in the decision-making process to move from Sacramento in winter, 2013, I once more raised the question to Dave's heart doctor. My query about Dave's mental functioning produced a similar result. By then I was seeing significant signs of neuropathology: loss of memory, strange gait, and redundant comments. I knew Dave needed help. I needed help. The situation was escalating beyond my capacity to deny. I finally convinced Dave to have an evaluation to see what we could learn. My feeling of victory was brief. I was dismayed to hear that because of limited resources in the neurology department of our health care provider, it would be six months before the assessment could be done. But then, this meant there was no great hurry.

The spouse may be the only person who sees certain behaviors. When trying to describe these anomalies they seem vague and just a little idiosyncratic, and their description may not communicate the serious and comprehensive level of impairment. When anecdotal behavior doesn't reveal a clear pattern, the spouse's concerns can be chalked up to over involvement. At this point, it would have made a huge difference if one of Dave's healthcare providers had suggested a referral to neurology.

I had become clear that we needed to move from Sacramento to the Bay Area in order to be closer to our family and had taken steps in that direction. At that logistical level I had acknowledged the seriousness of our situation. What I was not acknowledging was the impact on me and my need for help in understanding Dave's illness. Nor did I have any idea about how to go about getting more information. I thought I should know what to do. I didn't realize help was available, and that with more information about dementia, I could take better care of Dave and myself.

Dave pushed several times to get me to cancel the evaluation. I coaxed him into staying the course. Six months seemed like forever. The day finally arrived, and the picture became more complete. The "official" date, at least for Alzheimer's-like symptoms, was August 2013 when Dave was 81. It was at that point the neurology team at our Sacramento healthcare provider saw him. An MRI revealed bilateral shrinkage of the hippocampus (seat of memory functions in the brain) and other abnormalities. The index administered by a social worker showed that, not only was his memory faulty, but tracking and judgment were impaired. The evaluation validated my perceptions and indicated that Dave's condition was more advanced than I had thought. In hindsight the process had begun up to 15 years before this evaluation.

I have learned that diagnosis of Alzheimer's disease is tricky business. This condition can't be clearly diagnosed until there is an autopsy. It is the most prevalent dementia. Estimates say that 60 to 80 percent of people with dementia have Alzheimer's, but there are other dementias with both similar and different manifestations. Controversy swirls around possible causes and progress of the disease. There is no cure. Different theories account for what happens to people's brains as plaque and tangles* invade them; progress of the disease is unpredictable and differs from person to person. None of this motivated me to take Dave to a neurologist. And, strangely, I didn't delve into research about aging and dementia. I pushed the elephant as far out of the room as I could or just walked around it. Dementia couldn't happen to Dave.

Cardiac symptoms began to appear. On January 28, 2014, six months after we had the results of the first neurological evaluation, we were walking with a friend on the levee by the American River in Sacramento. Dave fainted. It was after a four-mile walk, which was more than we had intended. He was shaky and unsteady but was able to get up. He managed to maneuver his way up and over the levee, and he butt-walked down the steep embankment on the other side. By then we had rented an apartment in Walnut Creek, and we drove back there. We had agreed that if he didn't feel better, we would go to the hospital. We diagnosed his dizziness as the result of dehydration. We returned to the apartment and he rested for a while. He was tired, but not dizzy, and we were both relieved.

A few weeks later, on March 4, 2014, Dave awakened feeling unwell, and we went to the emergency room. He reported vague symptoms including dizziness and pressure in his chest. His description kept changing. He would say he had pain and then deny it. Yes, he was short of breath, No, he was breathing well. We had arrived at the emergency room around 10:00 A. M. and left at 4:00 P. M. with no new information.

Incidents like this one made it easy for me to doubt my judgment about what was serious and what wasn't. Did I overreact by going to the emergency room? Did I underreact by not going to the hospital when he fainted? Were Dave's symptoms real or did he imagine them?

Oddly enough, for a little stretch of time life was good. In mid-March, 2014, we had a bit of a break. We went to Scottsdale, Arizona, with friends, staying at a beautiful vacation rental in the desert and enjoyed our time together. While there, we attended two major league baseball games (spring training), walked through Desert Botanical Gardens filled with Dale Chihuly's magical glass works, and visited the Heard Museum in Phoenix. Desert air, blue skies, and good friends made for a sweet trip. Thank goodness we ventured forth, and no medical events marred our respite.

This time of normalcy made it easy to backslide into denial and doubt the severity of our circumstances. Maybe everything would be just fine. Not much fun, but not lethal. Life moved along well enough, although things I had always taken for granted like clear communication, empathy, energy for planning and creating next steps were blurring or slipping away. I could no longer rely on Dave to go to the grocery store and shop for supper, let alone plan what that was going to be, come home, prepare, and serve it. Life appeared normal, but it wasn't. His heart condition was more measureable and real than the dementia.

Dementia doesn't happen in a vacuum. While Dave's psychological slippage occurred, wear and tear of physical aging for both of us coincided. I see the loss of my partner to dementia as not only the loss of the relationship with him, but as the loss of a major part of myself. Even though in some ways this concept makes perfect sense and is easily identifiable, it is difficult to put into words.

"The people we most love do become a physical part of us, ingrained in our synapses, in the pathways where memories are created," Meghan O'Rourke states in her magnificent memoir of loss, *The Long Goodbye*.* And, certainly associations to memories of our loved ones trigger psychological and physical responses that affect our moods and sense of wellbeing.

We see ourselves, or parts of ourselves in our partners as they are reflected to us. A psychological term for this mirroring process is "self-reflecting other" * a construct from intersubjective-systems theory* that is relevant here.

You have probably noticed that you have a particular identifiable energy or feeling when you are with your partner or another important person in your life. In a good situation, that could be a sense of safety or self-confidence, high energy, and curiosity. According to the idea of the *self-reflecting other* some of this has to do with the way you are seeing yourself in the other person and the way that person reflects those parts to you. Different people, or for that matter the same person at different times, reflect different parts of ourselves. Only with a certain person do you feel this particular way. With another friend or with someone you don't like, you might feel like a (slightly) different person.

This is gross oversimplification of a deeply complex theory about which volumes have been written. The theory is subtle and complex. Because describing an emotional response is a little like trying to describe music or the touch of wind on your face, descriptions of how this theory works get so complicated they are often close to undecipherable. It seems worth mentioning, though, because it is a way of comprehending the depth of loss as dementia of whatever strain erodes a partner's personality. We not only lose the partner, we lose a reflection of ourselves in that person.

When I was with Dave I felt safe and like a good, competent, lovable person. Those were qualities he saw in me (and I in him), and I felt comfortable and at ease. As he faded, I was increasingly on my own making big life decisions, including those about his wellbeing. I missed the reassurance in his presence and had expanded room for anxiety and self-doubt.

In addition to what must have been the advent of Alzheimer's, Dave was beginning to have a significant hearing loss, which had gone undetected for some time. This guy was accomplished at appearing to understand what was going on around him. Since he was a quiet person and didn't always respond to a comment or volunteer one, it is hard to know how much he had been missing and for how long.

I retired from our psychology practice in 1998, four years after Dave did. I realized that spending time with him at home as well as in other settings was becoming more and more tedious. When we met new people, he invariably launched into stories about his abusive father, about his childhood and adolescence, and about his brief life in the military. Then he might reminisce about his athletic endeavors. He wasn't engaging in new activities or finding ways to entertain himself other than reading Spanish or watching sports. He spent his time working in the backyard, doing laundry or cleaning the house, and he seemed happy with this lifestyle. Since it worked for me, and he seemed content, it didn't occur to me to question the meaning of this retreat into domesticity or see it as a symptom of illness.

In the spring when it was time to buy new plants for the garden, Dave would count each of the big pots we had around the yard and make sure we bought exactly the right number of tiny plants, as if it were necessary to be precise. This seemed odd to me and different from the way I had known him in the past. Along with many other signs of something being not quite right, I let it slide. My response was to feel impatient and critical of this meticulous approach and then shrug. "Oh what the hell! What difference does it make?"

Dave was diagnosed with "Alzheimer's-like" symptoms in 2013, but long before that, I had uncomfortable feelings that something was off. It wasn't just that we were both retired and living at home. I've heard other older couples discuss issues related to an abundance of together time and how they would get in each other's way. But this was more than lack of space. Dave wasn't making sense of movies or tracking personal relationships. He was having trouble driving. At one point when he was navigating and I was driving, I was shaken to see that he was holding the map upside down. If I made a joke, he often didn't get it and would come back with some very literal response.

I assumed increasing responsibility for life's business and tried to cover in a way that preserved his self-esteem.

Dave knew something was wrong and that he was suffering from short-term memory loss. I overheard him tell a friend that he had a little dyslexia. I was shocked to hear this sophisticated diagnostician describe his failing memory with a term that applied to a reading disorder. He would talk about his memory loss as a normal part of aging with no awareness of the progressive nature of Alzheimer's. And, in fact, the creeping progress of his disease over decades had not been dramatic. He referred to his lousy memory, often noting that once he had a photographic memory but no more. Then he went on to the next thing.

Dave has never wanted to be a burden to me, and that has remained his central goal in life. I have been fortunate that he embraced this mantra and that his core kindness remained intact. There was no way I could tell him how his illness impacted my life. He couldn't do anything more than he has done to manage his side of our life together.

My hope is to describe how it feels to live an "as if" life with what remained of my beloved husband and the skeleton of our love.

CHAPTER 5

The Clamp

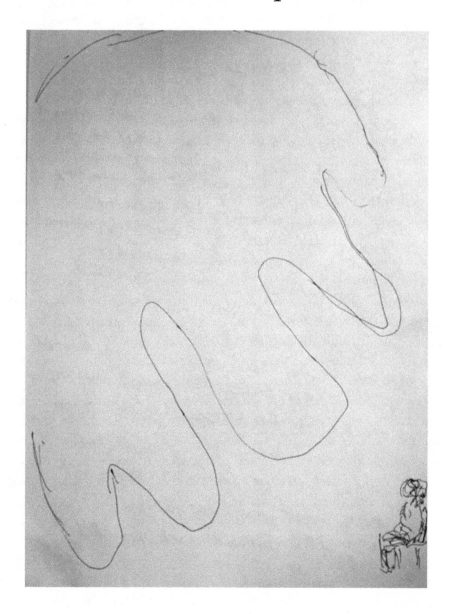

Black fog fingers stretching from a concave claw curled around my life and choked my spirit. While I was trying to absorb the meaning of Dave's terrible, terminal disease, I simmered, chafing against its reality. I couldn't define or validate my angst. I wondered if I was contributing to my ever-present low-grade distress, feeling whiny, deprived, angry, and resentful, by having unrealistic expectations for my life at this stage. More through imagery than words, I came up with language to describe what confined me: *The Clamp.*

The main reason I began writing this book was to come to terms with what I experienced on a daily basis. I had no road map or role model. Much of what I read or heard from others didn't fit my philosophy or value system. I thought if I could clearly describe my reactions to things, I could create better strategies for managing them. My approach had been to focus on logistics and numb out or attempt to transcend my feelings. Although that worked to a point, I could feel myself fading and shrinking.

I thought *The Clamp* was only in my mind, my bad attitude that I should overcome. I began to recognize it was more than that. There were real reasons I overreacted to seemingly unimportant disappointments and limitations. I was under assault without acknowledging my vulnerability in a life-changing situation.

I knew that if I could link vague, disturbing feelings to something in the observable world that agitated me, rather than attributing them to the overall situation, I could get better at managing them. For instance, if I felt inordinately sad and mad because of some change in plans, I learned to say, "This is where I am in my life, and my schedule is out of my control. This is part of life as a caregiver, and that's what I am. My true friends will understand; we will make another plan!" Then I could let go and move on. This was an improvement over berating myself for getting upset or thinking a better person would not feel depleted and hopeless.

My energy shifted from free-floating anxiety and depression to feeling more grounded and confident when I began to understand the power and structure of *The Clamp.* I could begin to cope with each of *The Clamp's* features rather than collapsing beneath the overwhelming undefined mass. I found these attempts to define *The Clamp* in my journal dated June 2016: "Life feels surreal. I can't get grounded and stay in my own groove. Pathos and yearning weigh me down. I could cry and cry and cry. I keep visualizing a dense presence composed of these layers:

- Negativity and anxiety emanating from Dave
- Feelings that I ought to be able to do this better
- Low energy
- Indecisiveness about what to do
- Unpredictability, my difficulty staying in the moment
- Dread
- Uncertainty about my health and longevity

Clarifying the reality of my situation allowed me to relinquish an old habit of self-blame that had crept back into my life.

I'm over-simplifying here, but I hope you get the gist of the process. When we know what we're dealing with emotionally, we can take steps to change or avoid the behavior or the situation. The problem for me was that I had such a hard time clarifying what made me feel unreasonably negative and constricted. My crashes and disappointments seemed out of proportion to the events that triggered them. I was in denial about how bad things were. My reactions were part of my much-needed wake-up call.

Shifting my role from partner to caregiver was crazy-making because in the beginning, many clues were subliminal. This drawn-out alteration was even more toxic because I didn't want to feel what I was feeling. I couldn't admit my angry and resentful feelings even to myself. Although I was a trained observer of emotion and behavior, experience had to stockpile before I could visualize and describe *The Clamp*. My mind struggled for words and images in an ongoing, looping conversation with myself.

As its definition emerged, I understood that *The Clamp* was a complex network of feelings. It was my self-defeating emotional response to being me in this increasingly difficult, ill-defined situation that I didn't want to be in. I began to devise language to describe this constellation of feelings. Something weighty was on top of me, clamping me down. I couldn't move around in my world. I had a hard time breathing and felt like I had no core, only expressed surface reactions to what was happening to me. Sometimes I realized that I had been spending time sitting, staring into space, unable or unwilling to move.

The Clamp's early calling cards were just little things. For example, one rainy Sunday our newspaper landed in a puddle and was waterlogged. Dave proposed lighting the barbeque grill to dry it out. He wasn't joking. What if he did something like that while I was at the grocery store? As much as I didn't want to accept this new reality, it was unsafe to leave

Dave at home unattended. I was clamped in place. I had to stay home just to maintain basic safety and status quo.

When I attempted to sort through my strong reactions to interrupted plans and disappointments, just for my own comprehension, *The Clamp* bloomed in my imagery. I could see the amorphous dark mist that shrouded me psychologically and held me hostage while the visible evidence of my life misrepresented what it felt like to be me.

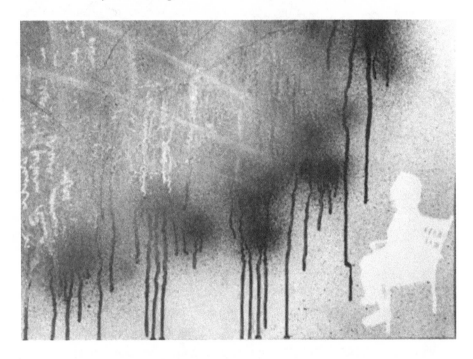

Because *The Clamp* seemed formless and all-encompassing, words failed me. I turned to drawing and painting, nonverbal media for nonverbal experience. The art was not pretty, but it began to illustrate my feelings of being confined and held down. I felt immobilized in the path of oncoming doom.

If you are nostalgic about the late 60's and early 70's, you might remember Ram Dass, (Richard Alpert, a Harvard professor and spiritual leader in the Age of Aquarius) and his book, *Be Here Now**. The idea of living in the present had made sense to me from the time I first heard about it, but in my caregiver role, I began to understand it as a necessity, a tool for survival. I needed to quiet the part of myself that thrived on plans and anticipation, another chink in my ways of feeling alive.

Nonetheless, our capacities to remember and to anticipate are important aspects of our selves and shouldn't be abandoned. The problem is that in fluid situations too much reliance on the past and the future creates frustration. "Be here now!" promotes focus on the present and allows us to benefit from what is before us rather than distracting ourselves with how it was or how it ought to be. "How are you?" people asked as a standard greeting. I couldn't answer this question, other than to say, "Fine," which says nothing. Actually, author Louise Penny's definition* in her novel *Fatal Grace*, fits beautifully here. "I'm FINE. Fucked up, Insecure, Neurotic and Egotistical," but that was more than I wanted to share most of the time. I could give no simple, authentic answer to the question.

I knew *The Clamp* was actually in me, not taking up space in my living room, although it might as well have been sprawled on the sofa. I couldn't move freely at home or in life. I felt constrained everywhere. In fact, to a limited extent, I had some mobility and was taking care of business, making art, taking walks, and practicing Qigong. Accomplishing this level of self care required commitment and determination, and sometimes, I just couldn't do it.

Scary as it was, the image of *The Clamp* helped me because it gave form and a name to my vague, contorted situation. It embodied a profound sense of loss, loneliness, and deprivation. After many years of therapy confronting and relinquishing my co-dependent* style, I found myself in a situation where I literally needed to re-enter that realm and guess as well as I could what Dave needed and do my best to provide it for him. Thinking for two certainly was more difficult than making one's way in the world independently.

The Clamp felt a little like other confining experiences I have had.

Journal entry: March 16, 2016

Sometimes when I am in airports waiting for a delayed flight or stuck at the gate for one reason or another, I sense that the air is filled with an invisible gel that inhibits movement, creative thinking or interesting activity. Even reading whatever I jammed in my carry-on for just such occasions seems superfluous. Options are all around but inaccessible, grayed out to me. I look at the other inhabitants, and except for an occasional child attempting to disrupt the goo, my compatriots stare into space, doze or appear sedated.

Life was normal in many ways. We had adequate resources: a comfortable place to live, a good-enough car, money for ongoing expenses and a few perks, computers, art supplies, money for caregivers, the necessities of life. But life was flat. Home was a terminal, a holding space. Going places with Dave was mobile caregiving. Going by myself or with others required significant pre-planning and funding for care providers. Unlike finding caregivers for pets, or even children, people who do elder care need special qualifications regarding elder-related health and safety interventions, in addition to the ability to relate to a particular individual who may not be happy to see them.

Talking with friends who were also taking care of spouses with dementia, I felt validated when I heard that their struggles with describing their reactions to the ongoing stress were just as poorly defined as mine were. We all knew we were stressed, but how could small events like repeated questions, disorganization, or misplaced items evoke such strong reactions? And, how could we describe the need for chronic containment in any way that someone who wasn't in the network could understand? I knew that my situation was mild compared to those who were dealing with incontinent, combatant, hallucinating and/or wandering partners. But, it was still me who was feeling empty, agitated, and overwhelmed.

Major aspects of my caregiver's job were visible, but those activities which devoured large bites of my time pie, weren't. Hence, *The Clamp*. This was something different. It was an emotional straightjacket, a foot on the chest, a smudged lens for the future, and an ever-present fuzzy membrane muting the sounds of joyful living.

I knew depression from both sides of the therapist's chair. *The Clamp* shared some of its qualities, but wasn't exactly the big D. It was waking up in the morning with a feeling of dread, looking at a day filled with administrivia while knowing that scheduling something enjoyable didn't guarantee bringing that event to life. It was going through the motions of helping Dave get ready to go somewhere in the car with me. I had become expert at repeating plans several times in clear, concrete sentences, sounding upbeat and accepting, remembering to avoid having "the tone" although it was the nth time I had said the same thing. I didn't always succeed. It's like parenting a toddler, but this one would require more attention over time, not less.

As an adult, I became acquainted with authenticity and learned to be more honest with others and myself which, at times, felt like peeling back my skin. Under *The Clamp* I found I had returned to acting mode where, no matter how I felt, I was to remain calm, upbeat, and encouraging. I thought of mean retorts to the advice given to Alzheimer's caregivers: "Be calm."

"You try it!" I would think. Or, "I have been calm for a whole week, and now I want to scream!!!"

A scene from my journal, March 2016, reminds me of the way I learned to manage situations that threatened to disrupt my carefully laid plans.

All week I have been thinking about today as my retreat day. I had plenty of sleep last night. It's a beautiful day! Dave came out of the bedroom. When I asked him how he was, he said "good." Then he said, "not so good. I might be a little short of breath. I think I shouldn't go to class."

"You may have some symptoms of bronchitis," I said. "You were coughing in the night."

He says again how bad he felt about my having to move to the couch in the night. "I don't want to be such a – and he moves his hands in front of him in claw-like down-pressing motion. Maybe I should go to a...someplace..."

I reassured him that he was doing just fine, and that I was doing just fine. I suggested that he go back to bed, that this has happened several times before and that possibly he would wake up in an hour and feel better. He took cold packs from the fridge to place on the nipple that harbored pain from shingles he had a year before and headed for bed.

As Dave inadvertently made the eerie rendition of The Clamp with his hand movements, I felt guilty and almost reeled. He executed the move perfectly, and one part of me wanted to scream, "That is exactly how I feel!" I could have said many things that would have helped us both down the road, like, "We will try out having you stay in a different place in a month when I go to New York, and we can see how it feels," or "It could happen that some day it will be necessary for you to live someplace else, but for now, we are doing well," but no. I freaked out and missed the opportunity. "Fine. We're doing fine."

I wondered if he had been reading my journal or the notes that I had been taking. Dave's sixth sense and intuition had blunted in recent times, but that was a part of him that had initially attracted me. He was highly intuitive and sensitive to the vibes around him, a capacity that served him well as a therapist and a partner. Remnants of that sensitivity remained, but not enough for me to rely on for genuine give and take in our relationship.

After all that, Dave got up, dressed, and went off to his day at Lamorinda Adult Respite Center, (LARC) which he calls "Late Adult Recreation Center." The R word is really Respite – for him or for me? Or for both of us? But Recreation worked for him. LARC is a program for people with dementia, housed and supported by the Holy Shepherd Lutheran Church in Orinda, California. It is designed for 15 participants, and there are three facilitators who conduct a variety of activities specifically suited to their clientele. Exercise, brain games, crafts, and live music are part of each day's program. Participants may attend from one to five days a week for the four-hour sessions. There is always a waiting list.

Did Dave remember our earlier conversation? I don't know. I did. By the time the driver picked Dave up to go to the respite program, I felt like I had worked an eight-hour day, and my plans were spiraling toward a nap on the couch rather than any of the other projects I had planned.

From what I have been able to discern, my primary reactions, conscious and unconscious, that empower *The Clamp*, are:

- Concern for Dave's well-being, but my inability to be on duty 24/7
- My desire to protect his self esteem while appearing to carry on life as usual
- Acting upbeat while feeling sad and/or angry
- GUILT
- Stress
- Fear of the unknown
- Fear of criticism and rejection
- Fear of doing the wrong thing
- Confusion/disorientation
- Resentment
- Deep sense of loss

Finally, I was able to ask myself the question behind the power of *The Clamp*. Why does an able-bodied woman with zest for life become the caregiver for a partner who is just getting by and has limited mobility and comprehension? I fully accepted responsible for making sure that he had good care, but did it need to be hand delivered by me? We were no longer lovers, business partners, parents, and adventurers. Romantic love and adoration had melded into caring and concern. I felt responsible for Dave's well-being with no expectation that he would contribute to mine.

When I married Dave, I didn't say, "…until death do us part," although surely it was implied. I'd already abandoned my first marriage. It wasn't exactly that. Dave had been a wonderful partner, and I wanted to treat him fairly. What did that mean? I had said to my daughters, "If I get like Dave, put me somewhere!" And, he had verbalized as much to me.

The problem was that I knew Dave well. He wanted to do the right thing, and he was very, very attached and dependent on me. I would later be proven wrong, but I was afraid that moving him to assisted living would precipitate a big decline, and I would feel worse than I already did, not to mention what that would mean for him.

Aha. Here is my personal understanding of how I gave power and reacted strongly to *The Clamp*: I was dying to have my own life, and I was too afraid, guilty, uncertain, and needy of approval to make the moves that would drastically change life for both Dave and me.

What a hard pill to swallow! At least the true nature of my dilemma, over a very long time, had become vividly clear to me. Painful as it was, clarity was a relief. I was beginning to grasp the big picture, and I couldn't erase that vision. The thought of living the rest of my life in the grip of *The Clamp* was too miserable to contemplate. There was a way to alleviate at least some of the pain in my life by making a series of major life changes such as moving Dave to assisted living, unthinkable as that seemed to me. I needed to marshal my courage, clarify whose disapproval I dreaded, and deal with those people directly or set aside that outdated fear. If I could accomplish these steps, I predicted my stress level would decline, and I would be able to reclaim myself. I needed more help.

Dave could do nothing to make the situation better. It was up to me. I could dismantle *The Clamp*.

Your definition of *The Clamp*, or whatever you choose to call it, may be partly or entirely different from mine. I urge you to look deep and sort through its complexity until you become clear about its components. Clarity is likely to come in stages as layers melt away, rather than in one huge aha! Each revelation helps.

As I defined and acknowledged *The Clamp,* I was able to comprehend my choices more clearly.

I had new sets of decisions to make.

CHAPTER 6

Watershed – Time to Move
2011 – 2013

When our grandson, Spencer Ginn, was born in late 2007, Dave and I began making weekly trips, driving 80 miles from Sacramento to Walnut Creek, to see him and to offer whatever help we could to his parents, our daughter Karen and her husband. We became overly familiar with that Highway 80 corridor and also began to learn our way around Walnut Creek. Sometimes we added another 80 miles to visit our daughter Erica and her husband Rex in Santa Cruz.

By late 2012, as we made our weekly trips to Walnut Creek, I began to think about finding a landing pad of our own in the area in order to have space, a pied-à-terre, in order to avoid inconveniencing Karen's family by needing to stay all night with them when we were in the area. If we had our own space, we could stay two or three days at a time and enjoy the Bay Area. I wanted to be part of Spencer's young life, but…

Dave resisted the idea of a small second residence and could see no reason for adding the expense. I too was concerned about our budget. I had done the math, though, and figured we could manage this project. Engaging him in the nuts and bolts of budget negotiation would not be productive because his ideas about the cost of things were severely outdated. His rock-solid resistance to change felt impenetrable to me. He had lost his willingness to engage in new adventures and was focused on staying put. He loved his house, yard, and pool, and that is where he wanted to stay.

As long as I believed I was making progress toward dealing with our lives and that a significant portion of my time and energy was productive and meaningful to me, I could do my caregiving job and make the best of our situation. During this period, though, Dave's needs were escalating, and I began to feel overwhelmed, a terrible feeling that I couldn't shake. Dread awakened with me in the morning, and I would think, "Another day of Dave." I wanted to cover up my head and go back to sleep. I remembered times in my life when I had been depressed, and I absolutely did not want to revisit that experience.

I walked a thin line, trying to win Dave's emotional consent to make big life changes without raising his wall of resistance. When I had heard others with compromised family members struggling with decisions about letting go of the family home or other familiar surroundings, I wanted to say, "Well, why don't you just tell him?" Now, I know why. It's harder than it looks. Proposing a major life change to a person who is anxious and having trouble remembering and tracking is one of the most challenging steps in the whole caregiving management journey. I appreciate that it is next to impossible to understand or view this incremental process with continuing patience if you are not the one simmering in the stew.

I would embrace positive feelings when I had them and attempt to feel a semblance of control in my life, but that feeling was invariably interrupted. I began tracking the process and can now look back at excerpts from my journal and see how the walls continued to close in.

Journal entry Wednesday, January 5, 2011

I feel optimistic about this new year; I am ready to deal with "next steps" as the process unfolds. I have some things I want to accomplish – the biggest of which is the art show with Ruth in Grass Valley at summer solstice time. But, dealing with Dave's anxiety is a full time job. About the time I feel I am in my own groove, he goes off on a spin. I need to invent ways to respond to him and then re-center.

November 26, 2011

The biggest loss is the absence of give and take in our relationship. My own aging process (memory issues, aches and pains, difficulty with multi-tasking, screwing up little stuff) accompanies Dave's reduced memory and judgment, his difficulty with mobility and his neediness. The loss of companionship creates an expanding vacuum in my life. There's also the thing of being the person in charge of all logistical arrangements, although Dave happily does the lion's share of housework, yard, pool, etc.

July 21, 2012

What a time this has been – the summer of death – and life. I feel weighted and like I have had little contemplative time or space for reflection. Even though I had thought a move was becoming possible and realistic, I have once again relinquished the plan for the pied-à-terre in Walnut Creek. That makes me sad. I can tell it is just too much, logistically and financially. It seems important to be more conservative about spending. Creating another dwelling is out of the question.

September 26, 2012

From the perspective of a casual observer, I have the best life anyone could possibly want. But the truth is, I'm a caregiver. If I have enough space for myself, I do fine. If I have too much exposure to the same stories, oversimplified conversation, or when I feel Dave is instructing or talking down to me, I get agitated and then depressed. I can drop into instant, immobilizing depression, and I don't feel like doing anything, even reading. It happened Sunday, and I spent much of a beautiful day in the dumps, doing nothing.

By late 2012 I felt immobilized but was going through the motions of my life, wanting to make some kind of move toward changing our situation. I had yet to create a way to get Dave on board for a big life change. I found it nearly impossible to describe, let alone justify my state of immobility. I could see, hear and feel myself being squeezed, but, because Dave and I had always had such an equal partnership, I couldn't bring myself to the point of taking over and authoritatively making decisions about the next steps in our lives.

Something had to change. I couldn't keep shuffling one foot in front of the other without taking action to make a difference. Finally it occurred to me to engage the family in a conversation about what was happening in our lives. Rather than discussing our decisions piecemeal individually or with couples, I wanted everyone to be on the same page with information, input, and the creation of some kind of timeline. Even though I had tried to communicate what was going on, I had been protecting all of us from grasping the seriousness of the situation. When we were in family mode Dave was his usual jovial self. The girls were not seeing the truth of our impairment. The holidays were coming up, and I didn't think the conversation I hoped for would be holiday-friendly. I decided to wait until after the first of the year.

At this point, our adult children were mid-career professionals in the San Francisco Bay Area with demanding schedules and limited discretionary time. Each one of us is an independent, strong-willed, opinionated person, not necessarily in agreement on important life issues, but having an undercurrent of loyalty and love that connects us. Rarely, with the exception of holidays, because of schedules and geography, were we all together, and even coordinating a holiday gathering was tricky. Imposing on our family was the last thing Dave and I wanted to do. However, at this juncture in our lives I dearly wanted the family's awareness and help, and I hoped for everyone to be on board with whatever plan we could devise.

After a few revisions, I sent the following email to Erica, Rex, Karen and her husband:

January 6, 2013

I have mentioned to each of you that Dave and I are involved in planning for our future and for elder care possibilities in the years to come. We have had several constructive conversations about this and have some ideas about how we would like to proceed, which we want to share with you. Input from each of you is important to us as well. One step in this process that we would like very much is to meet as a family and discuss some general categories: 1) hopes for the future, 2) needs as we see them, 3) fears and challenges, 4) strategies for mutual support.

We know that scheduling is difficult and that your lives are busy beyond belief. I am floating this request in order to plan ahead. I assume that a weekend day is best for all concerned, so that is what I am suggesting. Dave and I are not limited to weekends. Will any of these dates work? February: 16, 17, or 23, 24?

We would love for you to come to our house if that seems to be the best plan. We could have the meeting in the afternoon and supper afterwards. We will provide childcare for Spencer for the meeting time. If it is more convenient to meet in Walnut Creek or Santa Cruz, that is fine with us as well. For this moment your agreement to the concept and a date that will work for all is what we are hoping for.
Love,
Mom and Dave

The dates I suggested were far enough in the future to allow for planning. I was pleasantly surprised when the proposed date of January 17, 2013, was agreed to, a month earlier than I had hoped would be possible.

I had shared the email with Dave and discussed the idea of the meeting with him. He was in agreement. We had finally discussed finding a pied-à-terre in Walnut Creek, but the proposal for a permanent move waited in the wings.

The family, including Dave, met at Karen's family home in Walnut Creek around their spacious dining table on January 17, 2013. Spencer floated in and out, doing a good job of entertaining himself and giving us room to do our work. Without coaching or prior discussion, Dave stepped up to chair the meeting, once again reaching into his grace for connection, to hold us together and bring tears to our eyes. We proceeded through the agenda. The mini-miracle of his donning his customary leader role in the midst of my desert of despair invited openness, cooperation and trust from everyone. Here's a summary of the outcome in the email I sent after the meeting.

January 28, 2013
Hi, All,

Again, our thanks to you all for making our meeting a priority and showing up in all ways. I feel very relieved and supported by all and actually excited about exploring some next steps rather than feeling dread. Of course I gave a lot of thought to the meeting ahead of time, in order to be as specific as possible about why this gathering was important to me. Below is the outline I prepared for myself, filled in with notes from the meeting and then a couple of comments Erica sent a while ago.

I quit taking notes about half way through the meeting, and I know I have forgotten some important things. Please fill them in for me, and send them back. Also, I am sending this out partially as a perception check. These notes are from my point of view. If you understood something different, please let me know.

And if, like Erica, something occurs to you after the meeting that you would like to have noted here, please add it in. This is a way to continue our dialogue. Dave and I are finding it useful to keep a book of agreements, a bit of a memory aid for discussions we have had and

*insights that have come to us. I'll store a copy of this treatise and any
additions or corrections there.*
Thank you!

Family gatherings are usually holidays or special occasions.
We needed a separate time to do business to be intentional about
life changes. Thanks to Rex for pointing this out. The notes below
are the ones I made in thinking about the meeting ahead of time.
Italics are responses or conversation in the meeting.

1. Hope for the future:

    Continue as we are as long as possible.

    Know when it is time to make a move to assisted living
    or some other environment.

    Plan to move to Walnut Creek area within two or three
    years.

    Become situated so that the uncertainties and challenges
    of aging are not overwhelming and more depressing than
    necessary.

    *Karen's husband asserted that grandparental presence for
    Spencer is important, as well as connection with the family.*

    *Healthcare availability in and near Rossmoor, a large elder
    community nearby, is plentiful.*

    *Need to be aware of high level of regulation in planned
    communities.*

    *Dave expressed strong preference for renting rather than
    buying property.*

    *Dave and Nina are going to develop a plan for a possible
    move starting now, with exploring options and collecting
    information about Rossmoor and other communities.*

    They will make a list of questions and concerns.

    *Karen volunteered to help with this process in the Walnut
    Creek area.*

    *From Erica: it you are thinking about moving and or
    downsizing, and on a two-year plan basically, would it be a
    good idea to start thinking about downsizing your art collection?
    Hard to do, I know.*

2. Needs as we see them now:

Phone and email contact.

Moral support for the changes I am experiencing and anticipating.

Ability to travel and not worry about what is happening at home.

Spending quality time with each family member.

Knowing when you need support or something from me.

Knowing when you prefer for me to mind my own business.

Continuing with my art life.

What is the best way to bring concerns up to an individual? Direct, personal conversation.

You all expressed that our moving closer would make contact easier for you.

Dave and I feel the same way.

If we do move, we do not expect that family will be at our beck and call. It is important to us to be assets rather than liabilities.

Dave and I understand because of our small house it is difficult to have guests. We will continue to be the "visitors" and/or provide hotel accommodations if you choose to visit Sacramento.

Rex expressed a wish for more connection with Spencer and the Ginns and is frustrated by time and distance constraints.

Erica suggested it would be a good idea to have Dave see some kind of specialist, geriatric doctor, a neurologist, or someone who deals with aging brain issues and that there might be medication that would help. It seems like the chiropractor helped as much as possible, especially with his neck range of motion, but the brain issue remains. (Dave will set up an appointment with his doctor to see about a referral.)

3. Fears and challenges:

As Dave's needs increase, my personal resources will be stretched and I will be impatient and grouchy.

As my capacities diminish, I will have a harder time sorting out what I need to do to take care of myself versus being supportive of Dave and others.

If I become incapacitated in some way, family responsibilities could be beyond me.

It is important to check out both logistics and the "feel" of a move before making an irreversible decision.

Leaving Sacramento would mean disconnecting, even with the support of social media, from our network that has evolved over four decades.

4.   Strategies for mutual support:

Continue with family celebrations, serial and collective.

Continue regular visits to family.

Keep communications open despite busy schedules and geographic separation.

Karen's husband offered to co-sign our mortgage if Dave and I choose to buy a new home.

Karen's husband offered safe storage for Erica and Karen's flood-damaged photographs, a topic that had been mentioned in part of our casual conversation.

Everyone made clear Dave and I should spend resources rather than saving them for inheritance purposes

We will meet again in about six months in Santa Cruz.

I'm proud to be part of this family!

Love,

Mom

Communication among family members continued after the meeting. I felt immensely relieved. We had taken a giant step, and everyone had the same information.

Follow up email to family: January 30, 2013
Dave and I had a substantial discussion right after I sent you the earlier email. He came in questioning the need for the evaluation. He said, "It sounds like you think I have dementia." I opened up the discussion further, saying, "Yes, that is true. Your perception is accurate." I feel like we arrived at a new level as I gave him behavioral examples and

*let him know that everyone is concerned, but that it's hard to talk to
him about it. No one wants to hurt his feelings.*

Organizing and following through with the meeting had been
stressful for me, requiring lots of energy and thought. It paid off. I
was in a much better place.

Journal entry: January 30, 2013
*This is definitely a time of transition in my life. The family meeting
was a watershed:*
1. *The family expressed strong support for our potential move to
   Walnut Creek area, including support for a two-year timeline.*
2. *Karen's husband's strong invitation to us to be part of Spencer's
   life and their life was emotionally supportive in a way I did not
   anticipate.*
3. *Dave's mental challenges are now in the open, especially
   following his question this morning. "It sounds like Erica thinks
   I have dementia?"*
4. *I feel very supported and understood, not as alone and
   overwhelmed as before.*
5. *I believe a move to the Bay Area is a step toward something
   desirable, not just loss.*

This labor-intensive, systematic, and inclusive process required
reflection, planning, and the participation of all family members.
Summarized here, it seems fairly straightforward, pedestrian even, but
that isn't how it felt to me when I was in it. I hadn't known how people
would react to my requests or even whether we would be able to schedule
the meeting. I couldn't have predicted how Dave would respond to any
parts of it, or whether I had the capacity and stamina to carry through
whatever plan we created.

The outcome made the stress and effort well worthwhile. I was
deeply touched by everyone's heartfelt participation and willingness
to engage. As a psychotherapist who had spent years helping others
embrace authentic communication, in addition to doing the same
myself, I had been troubled by the necessity to be subversive about my
actions regarding moving from Sacramento.

Dementia patients don't do well with change or open-ended plans. I understood it was unwise to open a big list of move-related uncertainties to Dave's scrutiny. My process was slow and strategic. With the family's cooperation and involvement we were able to include Dave in such a way that he could comprehend and agree with the necessary steps. As I had seen him do before, Dave embraced the process and within a few weeks, was saying, "You know? It's time for a change. I'm looking forward to being able to spend more time near the girls." Knock me over with a feather…

January 17, 2013. Dave and I, with our family, had decided that it was time for us to have a foothold in the Bay Area, a place where we could spend time while visiting. I saw this step as a lead into a permanent move, as did the family. It was a way to slide into a new environment without abruptly moving the household. Karen found a perfect landing pad for us at the Ming Tree Apartments in Walnut Creek, a modest two-bedroom apartment downstairs at the corner of the complex, with a view of the pool and within walking distance of downtown.

Because this space was ostensibly our pied-à-terre, not a permanent residence, the Sacramento house remained intact. We furnished the little place with a combination of things we already had and a few inexpensive purchases. I had fun creating a shabby chic atmosphere, and it came together well since we had excess artwork, and an over-supply of linens and kitchen furnishings. On Washington's Birthday, 2013, just days after our family meeting, we signed a year's lease and over the next few weeks moved our assembled treasures into place. My journal reflects the shift.

Journal entry April 5, 2013
I have been frantically busy and have accomplished a lot, all that I hoped and more. I am very, very happy about getting moved into what we are calling the pied-à-terre and having it set up beautifully. Our financial situation is haunting me; I'm going to be optimistic.

April 18, 2013, Walnut Creek

The time here has been good. Dave is beginning to feel like he knows his way around. The trend is definitely in the right direction in that respect. I like it here. I love the apartment and feel that I can be comfortable here for a while.

I had accomplished this Bay Area partial move none too soon. Within the next six months I would start looking around for a more permanent set up. I was relieved that the partial move was in place, but, again, the next steps seemed overwhelming. As a permanent move to the Bay Area loomed in the future, the challenge of winning Dave's agreement was daunting to me.

A pied-à-terre was a manageable step.

The thought of selling our Breuner Avenue home and leaving Sacramento forever felt like hurling myself into space.

CHAPTER 7

FOR SALE!
2013 – 2016

"Well, Honey, because you have dementia, and we need to move closer to our daughters, I'm asking you to give up everything you're familiar with, including the house you love, and move to the Bay Area with me where we have no friends or connections other than our family. And, by the way, I'll be leaving people and places that are important to me."

Of course that isn't how I put it, but that was what needed to happen. I wish it could have been that simple. This chapter describes our family's approach to a wrenching life transition. Taking this step required acknowledging that life was no longer sustainable in its current form. It is easy for me to understand why families wait too long to make the move.

In 1976 Dave and I had purchased our home in Sacramento, near the university where we worked, and we lived there 37 years. In the year before the subject of moving came into the open, 2012, I shifted more deeply into my double life and focused on what it would take to accomplish a move logistically, financially, and emotionally. I went through the motions as always without embracing my inner life or living from that energy source. It reminded me of the time just before I left my first husband, behaving in one way and feeling another. ROBOWOMAN. Only this time Dave was leaving me. *The sacrifice of authenticity is one of many invisible losses familiar to caregivers of those with dementia, a prime example of how one loses oneself in the caregiver role.*

Even after he became willing to move, Dave didn't have the capacity to co-plan and orchestrate a move. His free-floating anxiety ballooned more and shrank less. If I shared anything about the steps involved in moving, his unending questions and confusion made me wish I hadn't.

Shifts in strategies or significant changes sent his blood pressure up and brought his apprehension into the open. He worried. Besides the strain that put on our relationship, I had dwindling room for my own fears and misgivings. Our partnership was dissolving.

I had wonderful support from my friend and wise woman Melissa, my partner in duplicity as she encouraged and supported me in clarifying and planning what needed to happen to accomplish a move. She was a sounding board throughout the process as I strategized and planned. She encouraged me to stick to the path when I felt like abandoning the whole idea.

Dave and I weren't alone in negotiating the currents of life, drifting in a canoe on an unpredictable body of water. Others occupied our craft as well. Whatever life decisions we made affected our family and vice versa. They were involved from a distance, though, and were only getting bits and pieces of the weather report at our house. Making things more difficult during this transitional time was Dave's uncanny capacity to maintain interpersonal contact with others with his ability to slide through conversations, which masked the damage that was occurring in his brain. Erica and Karen weren't picking up on the changes that were happening, although their husbands, who had very different relationships with Dave, were.

I knew that even after the decision to sell our house came together, the move would take time. In order to sell the property, we needed to update the kitchen, (a significant remodeling process), replace the backyard fence, and attend to other repair and maintenance issues. Melissa, my friend and confidante since graduate school, helped with kitchen project by coming up with a solid rationale: "Since the remodeling you have already done to the house is still fresh, this would be a good time to update your kitchen." Even though he could see no reason to change the design of the 1970's kitchen, Dave agreed with her logic. The plan was beginning to form, and I went to work finding resources to accomplish the remodel.

After Dave agreed to the kitchen remodel, I moved from making covert plans to asking for and sharing ideas and information as needed. Dave and I became a somewhat lopsided team moving forward rather than my feeling like a defensive, burdened wife dragging her unwilling husband into the unknown, but certainly dark, future.

The kitchen remodel ran concurrently with our move into the pied-à-terre in Walnut Creek. The job was a whirlwind affair and, ironically, was finished about the same time as the apartment became available. Fortunately, the company we hired to do the work accomplished the transformation just the way we wanted them to, on time and within budget. It was sad to leave the new layout before having a chance to enjoy it. My splurge was a magnificent red faucet for the kitchen sink. Definitely a case of little things for little minds, and I smiled every time I saw it.

Life felt upside down, and even though the pieces were coming together, the process jolted along unevenly. I could see the building blocks as my organizational mind mapped out steps for transition. If it were just me, it would be a lot of work, but not heart-wrenching. With Dave's confusion about time and space sequencing, wanting to help but not really able to, feeling disoriented and anxious, my job involved calmly providing support and containment for him while orchestrating the move.

Dave's neurological evaluation that I wrote about in Chapter 4 occurred at the same time we rented the apartment and remodeled the kitchen. New direction emerged as I was dismantling our familiar life pattern.

I became ROBOWOMAN. I gazed at the mountain of tasks ahead and feared I would collapse before I could reach the summit and maneuver my way down the other side. We needed to make the permanent move while Dave could handle the adjustment, and I still had the stamina to carry it through. I dreaded my own cardio evaluations that were coming up and hoped I would have no bad surprises. One of the few journal entries I found from this time said,

> *I see that I will be doing the move on my own and with resistance from Dave. I don't think there is any way he comprehends the seriousness of the situation, and, understandably, he is hanging onto Sacramento, all he knows, for dear life.*

True to form Dave did a complete 180. In mid-June, only three months after acquiring the apartment, Dave and I were talking about our little place, about Walnut Creek and how good it felt to be closer to the family, and he said, "We should consider selling the house and moving to Walnut Creek permanently." I should have put a red letter on this day or made a painting or written a symphony. But I didn't. I just felt overwhelmingly grateful.

From that moment, he joined the move and didn't look back. A few months later, as we were talking about how much we liked Walnut Creek, he said, "I was ready for a change." Moments like this when Dave seemed like his old self continued for the next year. They were little windows through the fog of his disease.

During the end of June and the first two weeks of July 2013, in the bloom of Sacramento summer, I orchestrated the completion of preparing the house for sale and moving our worldly goods to Walnut Creek into an apartment and a storage unit. Downsizing was a key word, and truckloads of art and art supplies, books, furniture, household goods, and other treasures went to new homes. With help from realtor, stager, contractor, floor refinisher, painter, landscaper, fence builders, pool guy, handy man, movers, apartment caretaker in Walnut Creek, Karen in particular and other family and friends, the miracle happened

The house we had lived in for nearly four decades and had remodeled from stem to stern sold in a week for our asking price, closing on August 27, 2013, our 40th wedding anniversary. By then we were permanent residents at the Walnut Creek apartment. We had the help of a storage unit for things that we didn't want to give away but couldn't fit in, and I had plans for finding an art studio as soon as the dust settled. We could be described as affluent refugees abandoning familiar surrounds in order to escape a form of isolation with Alzheimer's. As much as I hated leaving our friends, I felt that, in order to maintain contact and the mutual support of our family over the long haul, we needed to be geographically closer to them.

As I have learned about the dementia world, it is clear that this huge decision determined much of what would happen next and for the rest of our lives. When elders can't or won't choose to downsize and re-situate ourselves in order to access needed care, we abandon the possibility of making our own decisions. At some point, it becomes impossible or at least unwieldy for most people to maintain the container that was created for active mid-life. The decision-making then falls to family members, or we decline in our surroundings, overwhelmed by too many possessions and increasingly limited choices.

I was relieved and exhausted as I tackled post-move tasks: address changes, finding and securing health care, setting up utilities and other services, and the chains of details and sub-tasks attached to all of the above. Even though I had visited the East Bay Area for years, I had only learned my way around the territory adjacent to Karen's Walnut Creek home. Karen began educating me about shortcuts, traffic, services and restaurants. I dearly missed my friend network, walking buddies, and the ease of having lived in the same place for decades. Survival in a new, heavily populated environment with an impaired partner claimed my energy.

By September 1, 2013, we were members of the Kaiser health care system in Walnut Creek. Considering the centrality of medical issues as motivation for our move, I deeply appreciated the ease with which we changed healthcare systems. With one phone call and an hour completing forms we became part of a system that bundled our health services with the capacity to access digital records instantly from its many branches. The more challenging part was procuring our records from the Sacramento providers, some of whom required office visits and a waiting period to obtain paper documents for our medical histories and releases of information. The Kaiser hospital and medical offices were a mile from our new dwelling.

I found a good enough art and music studio a few blocks from the apartment and moved my art gear and vibraphone from the storage unit into that space. Although I had thought I could make it work, the spacious building in a big back yard never fit well for me. Having a day-sleeper in the house made music practice tricky, and the natural studio light was inadequate. I had a studio with poor lighting and limited music practice time. I had to go inside the main house to use the bathroom, a constraint I had seriously underestimated. It was, however, my own retreat space, and I spent time there every day.

I practiced playing my vibraphone and worked on several paintings in that spot, completing a 72" X 40" diptych, which was satisfying. It is a meditative piece more than anything, with a tree and each of a myriad squares containing many layers of careful painting. I listened to music and audio books while I worked. In those moments, I relaxed, regenerated, and felt like myself.

The tree image is based on a skeletal silver cedar along the trail to Lake Winnemucca near Carson Pass in the Sierra Nevada at or near 9,000 feet elevation. I have visited that tree several times and photographed it extensively. While I was working on the painting I was often reflecting on the conscious side of life and musing about the shadow side, the hidden reaches that are harder to access. The squares with their many transparent

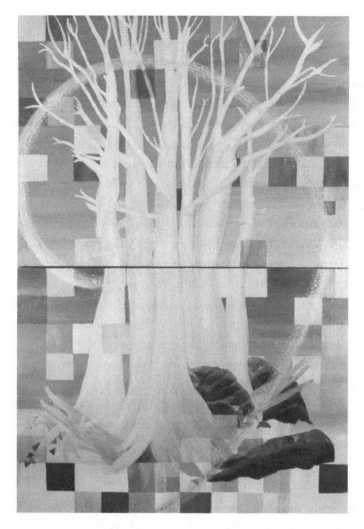

layers represent the ineffable or unseen dimensions that surround us. The Fibonacci spiral holds it all together. As I look at it years later, it feels like a truthful reflection of my life in this struggle.

Our apartment at the Ming Tree was secured as a pied-à-terre, not a permanent residence. It served its purpose beautifully, but with its not-so-hot studio, and encumbered storage unit, we knew we needed more space. My first plan was to rent another apartment in the complex, which could serve as a studio and guest room. For her own reasons, the owner would not agree to this unorthodox plan. Even though I waited for openings, she didn't relent. When I accepted the reality that my scheme wouldn't fly, I started looking for a new residence.

With Karen's help, again, despite the practically nonexistent availability rate in our area, we found suitable living space. Within three months, in May 2014, we occupied a dwelling she found for us within three miles of her home. This residence, technically a duplex, was, in reality, a well-designed house. It had a generous patio that served as outdoor dining space and art studio for up to nine months of the year. Breathing room!

My scheme to find a second apartment at the Ming Tree was born of a desperate desire to sidestep a second move. As life unfolded, we were much better off in the duplex than if my move-avoidance plan had worked. The second move was another mountain of work, but not as daunting as Move 1. This time we moved our previously downsized possessions from the apartment, Erica and Rex emptied the art studio, and, a couple months after the big move, with Karen's stalwart help, the storage room was empty. By then 2000 of my photographic slides and six linear feet of journals had been reduced to digits and existed electronically rather than in tangible form.

We lived in that comfortable duplex for two and half years. Dave did laundry, dishes, and cleaned. He sat in the recliner, gazed at TV, took his blood pressure, and snoozed.

The Clamp had developed physical manifestations over time. I had been having mild chest pains and other cardiac issues, which I tried to ignore, but when I had a chance to be away for a week, in August 2015, totally out of town, I noticed that I didn't have the symptoms that usually nudged me about my mortality. During the time away, several days had passed before it occurred to me that I had not awakened one time with heaviness or pain in my chest. This was a first in several months. I could no longer deny this evidence that the caregiver process was taking a serious toll on me, even though, by then, I had set up a functional help network and was determined it would succeed.

I understood that not one, but two moves would happen in the foreseeable future: Dave to assisted living, and I would find a smaller place, probably within walking distance of wherever he went. I wasn't sure when or how in the world I would ever find space, money, make lists, pack boxes, and get wheels on the road.

My heart ached.

I knew I was doing all that I could.

CHAPTER 8

Aging and Moving
in a Time of Dementia

Despite challenges, those of us who are old and getting older are the lucky ones who get to complain about aging. Friends and family are growing old, getting sick, and dying around us. It's that time of life.

As I dealt with Dave's heart condition, Alzheimer's, and other unnamed possibilities, I guessed and hoped for the best in making decisions, large and small. Along with orchestrating moves and trying to get a handle on the progress of Dave's illness, I discovered a variety of aging-related tasks that required time, energy, and decision-making. Some of these demanded daily attention, while others were more singular with long-term implications. And, then there was my own decline.

Medications: The details of keeping track of Dave's medication were front and center every day. Upon awakening, as a way of helping him stay oriented, I wrote the day, date, and schedule on a little white board attached to the front of the fridge. It was also necessary to monitor his meds: to keep the pillbox organized, make sure prescriptions were filled on time, and witness his ingestion of medications.

It was best if notes could be on the board and the pillbox filled and ready before Dave awakened in the morning. When these things weren't in order, he would become confused. If I stumbled from bed directly to the computer to record a dream or write in my journal, one of my ears would be oriented toward the hallway on alert for the sound of his footsteps.

Home Alone: Until sometime in 2015 Dave could be at home alone for an hour or two, but I wasn't comfortable being away for more than that. One of the ways I found time for myself was to get up early, check to be sure that he was OK, and then go for a walk. He usually slept until 9:30 A.M. I would leave a note saying where I was going and when I would return.

Hearing Loss: Fortunately, Dave's general health had been good over time because he stayed in shape and maintained healthy habits. Twenty years before, it had become apparent he had serious hearing loss, and we began a lengthy assessment for that. He willingly accepted the challenge of adjusting to hearing aids. When he was able to drive to his appointments and go to the hearing clinic, it wasn't a big deal. After we moved from Sacramento, every appointment required my involvement. The same with other medical issues that needed diagnosis or treatment, in addition to the major illnesses he was confronting. During our first months in Walnut Creek, it was a rare week when we were not at Kaiser for one or more appointments.

Pain Assessment with an Alzheimer's Patient: One of the added challenges I faced when Dave didn't feel well was his memory loss. If I asked him if the pain he complained about seemed about the same as it was three hours ago, there was no way he could answer the question. Because of his hearing issues and difficulty processing information, conversations with physicians usually had to go through me rather than his talking with them directly. This was especially true if I were relying on a telephone consultation to determine whether or not an office or hospital visit would be necessary.

The phone-in process had an added layer. Sometimes the nurse or physician, following protocol, would insist on talking with Dave. The notes clearly indicated that he had Alzheimer's and I was his authorized representative. It would then take at least double the time and frustration to assemble a plan for whatever the next steps might be. Because of his hearing issues, I had to advocate for him and advocate for someone to listen to me. Lots of repetitions were required, and tracking and memory challenges clouded his understanding of both the questions and recommendations. If he misunderstood a recommendation, which wasn't unusual, it would take patience, compassionate explanation, and tactful repetition to redirect effectively.

Palliative Care*: Through the Alzheimer's support group associated with LARC, I learned about the Palliative Care Department at Kaiser. Even though this Department was associated with Oncology and mainly dealt with cancer patients, it also welcomed Alzheimer's patients. In April 2014, Karen, Erica, Dave, and I met with a doctor in the Palliative Care unit and her teammates to establish a relationship with this department. For the first time I began to feel as if someone had the means to coordinate the big picture and deal with Dave as a whole person and help us as a family system in regard to his dementia.

Signing on with the Palliative Care Department meant that I could consult with them about whether or not a hospital visit was necessary when Dave had symptoms of one kind or another – that is if the symptoms occurred between 9:00 A.M. and 5:00 P.M. on weekdays. It's surprising what a small portion of the health week those hours cover. Symptoms arrive at other times: Friday evening, Sunday morning, 3:00 A.M. on Tuesday. However, when the timing was outside office hours, someone on the Palliative Care team attended emergency room visits or other hospital stays. This provided tremendous support for both Dave and me about any decision making that might have been involved. Yes, we treat for a urinary tract infection (UTI). No, we do not do emergency heart surgery.

Also, it was reassuring to call the Palliative Care Team, when they were available, and have a professional say to me, "This sounds like a time to wait and see what happens two hours from now." I knew that if Dave were showing signs of heart attack or stroke, I would call 911. The professional input on non-critical occasions lifted some of the load from me.

The Caregiver's Health: Then came an uninvited opportunity to look at my own aging and mortality. I had a moment of clarity about the importance of doing the things that are meaningful to me instead of *waiting*.

In April 2016 I had gone to Kaiser for routine blood tests and a blood pressure check prior to my yearly physical. My heart rate was low: 44 beats per minute. I assumed it was because I had just finished walking and doing Qigong, but the nurse who took my vitals didn't buy my diagnosis. She told me to discuss it with my physician when I had my appointment. I acknowledged having had some weird pressure feelings and slight pain from time to time. She gave me the look and said, "…you know what to do."

In addition to having a really ugly sun damage spot frozen off my arm, I brought up the low heart rate item. My doctor said that would be OK if I were an athlete. I told her about walking and Qigong. She said, "No, I mean an athlete at the level of Lance Armstrong." I wasn't sure I liked her example, but I got the drift. She instantly referred me for an old-fashioned electrocardiogram (EKG), a stress test, and an echocardiogram, all of which I accomplished in that one visit.

While I was on the echocardiogram gurney (not looking at the screen) I had significant reflection time while the technician poked, prodded, and clicked the computer keys. The procedure took approximately 20 minutes. I'm thinking, What if I have something seriously wrong with my heart? I was saddened and scared by the idea of dying or being seriously disabled as a caregiver before I could fulfill my fantasies about life in the Bay Area.

My doctor prescribed a Holter heart monitor for me to wear for 24 hours. The Holter is a little recorder that has electrodes attached to wires and then your body. It offers up an extensive EKG, which reports cardiac activity or inactivity. The instrument can be concealed easily enough under bulky clothing.

I managed to look and act "normal" at home while wearing the Holter because discussing this with Dave would lead to questioning, repetitions of those questions and answers, and Dave's amplified anxiety. I was anxious about what the monitor was reporting and mildly uncomfortable. More uncomfortable though, was the deception. I still wasn't accustomed to hiding such things from Dave. How many times? 20? 50? I almost said something?

I was relieved when the outcome of the heart measures showed I was functional for that time but might need a pacemaker in the future.

When we had moved in 2013 downsizing took its toll. Life's logistics came forward with their demands, including the intangibles of approaching life's end: health care decisions, wills, and powers-of-attorney for financial and medical decisions. Even less observable were the emotional aspects of leaving the city where we had met, fallen in love, and lived for more than four decades. At the most practical level all the networks and systems we relied on had been in flux:

- Health care
- Transportation
- Financial services
- Familiar sources for shopping
- Legal status
- Help network
- Postal services
- Social life
- Entertainment venues
- Service installation/reconnections

Cutting and re-weaving each of these network threads added both logistical and emotional challenges. Paper trail took on new meaning. Dave and I led simple lives by today's standards and were no longer in business. Yet changing addresses, banking, healthcare, everything about automobiles, insurance, Internet, and phone services seemed endless. The nonmaterial facets of moving had been as numerous and time consuming as boxing up the pots and pans and exterminating dust bunnies. I had confidence the move would come together, but the decision was loaded with stress and loss.

Nonetheless, I was determined to grip a lifeline of fun and normality. For years Dave and I had attended *Songe d'été en musique* where we stayed with our friend Karen Davis at her farm in the Eastern Townships south of Quebec City. We enjoyed beautiful music played by our New York friends, who came to the area to create this midsummer music dream. The summer of our big move in 2013 had been no exception. We had plans to go and, with strong encouragement from our family and friends, we persevered. It was Dave's last trip to that sweet and magical place. Our friend, Rachel Guerrero, accompanied us and helped in many ways on the challenging but hugely rewarding journey.

Advanced Planning: With the change in healthcare came the questions of "Advanced Planning," a euphemism for deciding who is in charge of decision-making if you are in a life-and-death situation. Do you wish to be resuscitated if your heart stops? Just how do you want to die? We began this process of decision making with our attorney in Sacramento and finished it thanks to a workshop in the neurology department at Kaiser in Walnut Creek.

POLST*: Creating a Physician Orders for Life-Sustaining Treatment (POLST) brought me face to face with end-of-life issues. It's one thing to say, "I don't want any heroic measures." It's daunting to choose between 1) pull the plug if my brain will never work again, 2) pull the plug if my body will never work again, 3) pull the plug if both of the above are true, 4) do what you can to keep me comfortable and let me die, or 5) resuscitate no matter what. After going through this dress rehearsal for the final scene, I read a book that would have been helpful at the moment: *Being Mortal** by Atul Gawande, a surgeon who writes candidly about end-of-life issues. Read this book or one like it!

Legal Steps: With any condition that erases a person's ability to manage their own business and legal affairs, someone needs to be in charge. Attorneys who specialize in serving elderly clients can help with planning for the person's care. The Alzheimer's Association lists three key issues to address:*

- Options for health care decision making for the person with dementia
- Options for managing the person's personal care and property
- Possible coverage of long-term care services, including what is provided by Medicare, Medicaid, veteran benefits and other long-term care insurance

Working with an attorney who specializes in elder care can ultimately save time, money, and distress. I strongly recommend that you find a good one, as s/he can do many things that haven't even occurred to you. You don't know what you don't know, and that can cause so much stress. The Alzheimer's Association provides a checklist of items to bring to a first meeting with an attorney:

- Itemized list of assets (e.g., bank accounts, contents of safe deposit boxes, vehicles, real estate, etc.), including current value and the names listed as owners, account holders and beneficiaries
- Copies of all estate planning documents, including wills, trusts and powers of attorney
- Copies of all deeds to real estate
- Copies of recent income tax returns

- Life insurance policies and cash values of policies
- Long-term care insurance policies or benefits booklets
- Health insurance policies or benefits booklets
- Admission agreements to any health care facilities
- List of names, addresses and telephone numbers of those involved, including family members, domestic partners and caregivers, as well as financial planners and/or accountants

Concurrent with our move from Sacramento came the need to take over Dave's legal and financial decision-making, something I had dreaded having to approach. I couldn't predict whether he would agree with this step or whether he would protest. Because of his short-term memory loss and diminished judgment, he was no longer competent to carry on business, and I needed to have his Power of Attorney (POA)* in order to handle legal, financial, and medical issues as they occurred.

We updated our wills and took the necessary steps, including providing for Erica and Karen to have POA for me. Dave seemed to know what was going on in these conversations with our attorney and willingly signed documents to make the arrangements. I felt fortunate he was able to turn decision-making over to me in a cooperative manner. Almost immediately that POA came in handy for obtaining records and making financial and medical decisions. Accomplishing these legal changes took multiple trips to Sacramento and shuffling papers among family members to have them notarized after we had moved. I was relieved to mark this set of chores off the list and glad that I hadn't waited any longer.

Driving: The Alzheimer's plot unfolded in stages, each of which might have seemed innocuous in the beginning but intensified over time. Driving had become an issue between Dave and me. Dave's reaction times were slow and his decision-making at intersections had become increasingly impaired. Once he told me cars were coming toward us in the wrong lane as we were crossing a long suspension bridge that had a parallel span for oncoming traffic. Fortunately I was driving that time, but Dave remained adamant about his right to drive.

We had made the permanent move from Sacramento into the Ming Tree apartment in Walnut Creek in the spring of 2013. At that time I bought a different car and disposed of the two we had. We only had one space in the lot. Dave backed off his demands to drive, and he shifted by saying he had decided not to drive anymore. We went to the Department of Motor Vehicles (DMV) and procured an identification card that looked like a driver's license but wasn't. I became the sole driver. Subsequently, he began telling people that he realized that he was a danger on the road and decided to surrender his license. After years of struggle on this issue, I had a hard time refraining from snide comments and eye-rolling, but I managed.

Dave gave up driving, but he amped his participation as the virtual driver with infinite instructions to me on traffic, parking, road hazards, and speed limits. In my younger, less restrained years, I probably would have parked the car, thrown away the keys and summoned Uber if it had existed. At this stage, I only considered that rash act. I began sneaking off to the grocery store as needed without inviting him to come along. Anytime we both entered the car, my stomach hurt. When I heard people in the Alzheimer's support group talking about driving struggles with their loved ones, I broke out in a sweat. It was one of the most distressing steps in dealing with the illness because it is linked with an individual's identity and personal power. Handing over that driver's license is surrender. Even with the support of a physician and the DMV, fights occur, lies are told, and blame is infinite.

Money Management: Money management was another responsibility that finally landed on me. For years, Dave had paid the bills and handled our joint finances. We had individual checking accounts and a joint account for our household expenses. It was an arrangement that we liked, and I often recommended to couples in counseling. As I observed him having more and more trouble with the checkbook I had set up banking on line and arranged for most on-going bills to be paid automatically. Eventually even that wasn't enough.

One day I came home from downtown Walnut Creek to find Dave on the street in front of the duplex attempting to write a $400 check for a woman who was selling magazines. I was able to intervene. I didn't need any more information about the importance of removing him from money management. His good will had always had a direct line to his checkbook. Impaired judgment meant it was time to seal that outlet.

I took over all money management, leaving him with a small bit of cash for his wallet, a couple hundred dollars in a checking account and a credit card that was actually mine, but it had his name on it. I paid for dinner when we went out or for other things we did together. In an effort to preserve his dignity I mentioned that when I used the credit card I would get points toward airline miles.

Personal Safety: Erica and Rex came to visit bringing forms with block letters in red and white saying FILE OF LIFE, which they had picked up at an Alzheimer's Association workshop. These handy packets contained all the vital information that first responders need. They were attached to the fridge along with the white board containing the day's schedule, a list of caregivers and helpers, and a few photos of Spencer and other family on a rotating basis. The Physician Orders for Life-sustaining Treatment (POLSTS) were on file at Kaiser, and we had copies in the glove compartment of the car and in the buffet drawer.

Logistics, Geography, Shopping: The minor tasks of finding a lampshade, rain coat, or some other supply quickly, close by, with available parking, could no longer be mastered easily. Each chore could become a time-eating project while many others waited to be addressed. Getting around geographically, and learning ways to avoid traffic added to my learning curve.

Friends and Moving: Even though it took ages to coordinate the move, when the decision for permanence erupted, it was more like a volcanic spew than a river of decision. Our next-door neighbors didn't realize, until the moving truck was in the street, that we were leaving forever. In March 2013, the move had been an exploratory venture into the Bay Area. By May it was to be permanent. The neighbors thought we were still in pied-à-terre mode and would continue living in Sacramento until an undetermined future date.

My thought was that the Bay Area wasn't that far from Sacramento, and, with social media, it would be easy to stay in touch with important people in my life. I had been so focused on planning, organizing, and controlling the move I had pushed the centrality of my friend network to the back of my mind. I had good friendships in Sacramento that went back to the '70s, 40 years or more, and I couldn't let myself think about how much I would miss them. I closed my eyes and moved forward. I still miss them. I see a few of them from time to time, and I am grateful for that, but they are irreplaceable, and I yearn for our shared history and easy companionship.

Family: Karen helped me in more ways than I can count in finding resources and guiding me around our new hometown. She was upbeat and good company. Erica and Rex were solid supporters, helping whenever they could. Judy visited frequently, bringing her good will and support. Two or three other friends came to see us on a regular basis, and I would arrange to go to San Francisco or on some other day trip with them. Even though he had become increasingly less steady on his feet, Dave could still go for a walk and help with some of the things we needed to do.

The move had been a good decision. It felt wonderful to be in the same town with Karen and her family and closer to Erica and Rex. We became more involved with Spencer's life, which was pure joy. I began to enjoy a small bouquet of friends. I stayed in touch with my old ones in the usual long-distance ways, but that was less intimate and satisfying than going for a walk, out to lunch and a gallery, or having a party. Other than my big easel I didn't miss the carloads of clothing, household goods, furniture, art, and books we had given away. I was getting to know some people I liked, some of whom I hoped would become real friends.

My relationship with Dave had changed completely. Its original jellybean shape with two equal sides had slumped to a bloated figure 8 flattened on one side. Our mutual balanced love relationship had converted to one of caregiver and patient.

I was self-critical about my impatience and diminished sympathy. Please don't emulate this. I felt that I should be a bigger person, more capable of supporting my partner in his aging process. I was certain that if the tables were turned, he would be generous to me. Instead I saw him as a hypochondriac focused on his physical symptoms rather than getting at the source of his anxiety and dealing with it. He constantly wanted to help me, and he became overly solicitous. This is going to sound paranoid, and perhaps it is: I began to feel like I was under constant scrutiny. Dave seemed much more interested in my activities than he was in his own. He watched me carefully. If I had a crumb on my face or a loose hair on my shoulder, he helped me correct the flaw. He found or invented any excuse to help me. Now I understand these were manifestations of Alzheimer's, but as they evolved, I felt myself shrinking and wanting to run away.

We do what we can to maintain our equilibrium. Even though I'm not religious in any traditional sense, I began praying for *patience* and *compassion*. When I found myself wanting to scream or feared I might implode, I would breathe quietly but deeply to intone my silent mantra: Patience and compassion, patience and compassion, patience and compassion, please give me patience and compassion.

Journal entry: January 2013

In grade school, we had oversized wall clocks that clicked with each passing minute; I could see the big hand move until it finally clunked against the next number. I watched as the minutes stretched longer and longer until finally the click came that signaled the end of the period, and I could move. I learned to watch the clock and look like I was reading or doing my work. Seems like yesterday or a long, long time ago. And now I'm a clock-watcher all over again.

For me, picking up responsibility for every detail in another person's life felt like being pecked to death by a flock of ducks. No one peck is too painful, but there is no respite. Every moment holds a need or demand. Little room remains for one's own concerns, whether about aging or life in general. When I began having fantasies of driving to New York instead of going home, or of crashing the car, or getting sick in order to avoid dealing with my life, I knew I had to take stock and find the means to extricate us from impending entrapment in dual dementia. (See the movie *Iris,* 2001, starring Judith Dench and Kate Winslet.*) My need had moved beyond theoretical to life-threatening.

Later I understood I had seriously underestimated the changes that were happening with Dave. He was still kind, charming and supportive in certain ways, masking his memory loss and secret terror. My denial was slow to go. It is possible that Dave knew he was no longer capable and thus bought into my semi-invented reasons for the decisions I made. My job volume was bursting and the enrichment portion was dry. Despite whatever I was facing in my own life, I was a full-time caregiver. I had unintentionally joined a worldwide web without my explicit consent.

Welcome to the network.

CHAPTER 9

HELP!!

I needed help. Who doesn't in this caregiver role? What isn't obvious is how difficult that was to accomplish, especially in a new environment with no established social network.

Some family caregivers resist getting help on principle, feeling that doing so would be disrespectful to their loved one. That was not my problem. One way to look at this situation is to think about whether or not you would let a physician into your home if you had a serious illness. If the answer is yes, the next step might be less threatening. I had learned that being overwhelmed as a caregiver is serious.

Surely someplace in our neighborhood there were people who would love to come to our house and be a companion for Dave a couple hours at a time, which would make it comfortable for me to leave the house. I began asking around. Dave requested that his companion be a man. That narrowed the field by a factor of eight or more, but no worries. My search was yielding exactly zero results. I thought about our extended social network in Sacramento and yearned for similar contacts in Walnut Creek.

A friend in Sacramento happened to know of a caretaker who was tending a relative of hers in our area. That caretaker had a male cousin who might be available. Great! Except he was only available certain days and required a five-hour minimum at $20.00 per hour. He came to our house a few times and did an adequate job. When I first began learning about the cost of caretakers, I was dismayed. How could I pay someone $20 an hour so I could go for a walk or to the grocery store? That seemed surreal.

Then, one day our caregiver showed up when he wasn't scheduled, and another time he canceled at the last minute because he didn't have transportation. He got a job in another town and was less and less available. Some help should be better than no help, but my frustration soon outweighed the gain. I needed to establish a list of caregivers, and I was getting nowhere fast.

One of the great joys of retirement is having a flexible schedule. I began to get the drift that finding someone to stay with Dave meant I would need to schedule my time according to the caregiver's availability. I dropped "spontaneous" from my vocabulary. This was not an easy trade-off for me.

My vision of the caregiver process and the reality of having help were not on the same wavelength. My initial worry was about the expense and being vulnerable to an unknown person caring for Dave in our home. Dave understandably resisted the idea that someone needed to be with him when I was away. Companionship had to be arranged in some way that preserved his dignity. This is one of the biggest stumbling blocks for anyone who is attempting to arrange outside care. My approach was to say that I worried about his being alone in case of an emergency or something unpredictable happening. The helper didn't have to do much more than be present to respond in the event of an emergency. They also had to be trustworthy, dependable, and capable of making a connection with Dave.

By summer 2014 I felt more and more desperate. A woman I had seen walking in the neighborhood knocked on the door and said she was just stopping by to get acquainted. I invited her in because, I reasoned, she lived in the neighborhood and might know people who could help us. I blurted out to her that I was looking for caregivers for my husband who had early to midstage Alzheimer's.

"You need to talk with me," she said. "I've been doing elder care placement in this area for 40 years. That's my job."

Karen and I met with her shortly thereafter, and she helped in substantial ways, most importantly by recommending that Dave check out the possibility of attending Lamorinda Adult Respite Center (LARC).

At the time I didn't think there was a chance in the world that Dave would even consider attending a daycare program for people with dementia. This is a great example of my not seeing his level of impairment. How could I know that he would be thrilled to find a place where he could fit in without having to "perform"?

At the time, I was deeply engaged in preparing for an art show that I was going to hang in Oakland the first of February 2015. Come hell or high water, I desperately forged ahead, clinging to what seemed like "my life." Generously, Karen took over the project of exploring the respite program. She visited LARC and another daycare program nearby. She felt that LARC was a good place for Dave, "There are guys there who look like college professors," she said. "I think Dave will like it."

Karen initiated taking Dave for a test run at LARC and sat through enough of a session to see that he would be comfortable there for the rest of that day. The program operates from 11:00 A.M. to 3:00 P.M., daily, and participants can choose the number of days they want to attend. With Karen's help, Dave agreed to try it two days per week for one month. Karen took him to his first real session and sat through part of it. He LOVED it. I was thrilled and surprised. I was very glad to have been wrong. Other than needing to drive him back and forth, 20 minutes one way, my Tuesdays and Thursdays now had some breathing room, and Dave was engaged in something that he truly enjoyed.

The fact that Dave connected strongly to the LARC program was diagnostically significant, but I missed that part of it. The activities there were geared for people with dementia. He felt comfortable and entertained with that level of interaction. He could relax and didn't have to maintain any pretense of understanding things that were going right past him. I still wasn't getting it.

Support Group: Along with LARC came a support group of people whose loved ones (the term of choice for people with a dementia diagnosis) were in the program. This unfacilitated group met weekly in the same location as LARC but in a different part of the building. I began attending. Members had loved ones in all stages of dementia from just being diagnosed to deceased. Having been a professional group facilitator for years in different settings, I found it challenging to be a member of an unfacilitated support group, and I resisted urges and opportunities to take over and focus the discussion or move things along. With a little patience and respect, I learned that the folks in the group were doing a fine job of taking care of business.

The group tolerated me, and I felt at home and, well, supported. I began learning the ropes of the care system as well as many other things that are part of being a caregiver. Many group members had been through the fine-grinding caregiver mill and were willing to share their experience honestly and with compassion. I am forever grateful to these people, many of whom experienced deeper and darker times than I. I feel privileged to know these folks.

The greatest gift of the support group was meeting Joanie Forney, the wife of Dan, one of the LARC members who became Dave's good friend. Joanie and I formed a dynamic duo and supported each other as we took necessary actions to wend our way through the caregiver world and all that entailed. We encouraged and consulted each other regularly throughout the next few years as we faced similar challenges.

With LARC, I had secured from three to six hours per week of "free" time, depending on whether or not I attended the support group. That left lots of other time in which I still needed help at home. I decided to try the agency the consultant had suggested. One of the agency principals came to our house to evaluate us, and to see if we were a good fit for their program. We passed. They said they would try to find a male caregiver and asked if we would be willing to have a woman until they could. Here again, scheduling was an issue. Their employees wanted eight-hour shifts, the same day each week, at approximately $28.00 per hour, the agency rate. It would be next to impossible to do it any other way. Several different people came out over the next few months, but never a man.

Another agency did send a man who was a kind and competent person. He was also anxious. I could see that the fit wasn't good. He found another job just about the time I was going to let him go. I tried a couple of other guys from that agency who were adequate for a time or two, but not as ongoing contributors to our household.

Care provider agencies can be useful but the problems I have noticed made it difficult for me to maintain this form of help over a period of time. The agencies undoubtedly have high expenses. They pay their personnel low wages. The price tag for the client is high – around $30 an hour in 2015, usually with a minimum number of hours required on a regular schedule. While many dedicated people work for agencies, there are also many people who work there because it is entry level work and available. Training is minimal. If the usual care provider isn't available for some reason, another one is sent, which is confusing for people with dementia.

In addition to short periods of time for grocery shopping or errands, I desperately needed time to myself for occasional overnights or brief stretches away from home. I yearned for little trips with friends, attending art or writing workshops, or experiencing some change of scenery for a long weekend. I also craved time alone at home to paint, play music, or do nothing. Finding affordable care for this kind of respite seemed impossible.

In the summer of 2014, as much as I wanted to be there, I had been too overwhelmed to attend *Songe d'été en musique* in Canada and hang out with Karen Davis and our other friends. In 2015, my sister Judy agreed to accompany me to Canada. What about Dave's care while I was away? His well-being during my week-long absence depended on 100% reliability of whatever care plan I could patch together. The one I created involved family, friends, paid caregivers, and drivers. It also entailed making sure the house was supplied with food and other necessities and orienting helpers so it would be easy for them to find what they needed. Even with perfect intentions, careful planning and very responsible people, things could happen to rip the safety net.

By the time I completed the detailed plan for Dave's care I knew I would never again go through that process. I set up a calendar with the information for each day: instructions for whomever would be involved in at-home-care, LARC transportation, overnight stays, emergency instructions, and specifics about the house. I did the grocery shopping for a week. I kept in mind special needs of the caregivers as well as Dave.

If you glance through the schedule, it really doesn't look daunting until you get a little more data. Karen is our daughter who lives nearby and has a busy professional and family life. Steven was a caregiver from an agency. Our friend Rachel came from Sacramento to help out. Erica and Rex came from Santa Cruz, and Nora, Dave's sister came from St. Louis. We had six people involved, plus trips back and forth to LARC, listed on the schedule as "class." In addition someone had to pick Nora up at the airport and take her back there for her departure.

Thanks to this ensemble of friends and family who care deeply for Dave and me, Judy and I were able to make the trip. We had a wonderful time. Nothing disastrous happened while I was gone. I returned home feeling happy and renewed, and I knew more than ever that it was essential for me to get away from time to time. I needed to find another way to provide care for Dave in my absence.

In the support group I learned about various care options. One was to arrange for the loved one to stay at an assisted living facility in "respite care" for a predetermined period of time. Most places required at least two weeks. For the Long Island and Canadian music festivals in 2016, I decided to explore that possibility, and eventually it worked out. It was problematic that the facilities wouldn't know whether or not they had an opening until less than a week before departure time. To be eligible Dave needed a recent tuberculosis test and a physician's evaluation regarding his health status, mental capacity and needs for assistance. An interview by the nurse at the facility to determine his level of functioning and a "skin check" were parts of this as well.

Those were just the logistics. What about Dave and his feelings about entering an assisted living facility? What would that be like for him? Would it have a negative effect on him? I felt like I was asking a lot of him so I could go play with my friends.

On the other hand I needed to take care of myself, and it didn't make sense to give up my life and my needs while I still had capabilities. My low heart rate and murmurs indicating valve issues were not predictors of long life. I wanted to insert patches of joy and excitement in the here-and-now. Dave's stay in respite care would be time limited. I could do both to some degree: take care of Dave and take care of myself.

Journal note: August 30, 2016
> *I feel like the meanest person in the world*
> *But*
> *Why?*
> *Should a person who has zest for life*
> *Crawl into a cocoon*
> *To care*
> *For someone*
> *Who*
> *Does not know what day it is*
> *Can't find their way down the street*
> *Is happy being silly, doing trivial pursuit,*
> *And listening to popular music from 60 years ago?*

Fortunately, Dave's LARC friend Dan had stayed previously at the assisted living place we were looking at. His experience had been better than okay. He and Dave could be at the facility at the same time and would also attend LARC during the week I was gone. This arrangement was at least 10 times easier than the previous year's at-home plan, and it ended up being less financially daunting than the complex plan I had created for in-home care. We went through the evaluations and prepared as if it were going to happen. Dave embraced the idea with the thought that he would be helping me out, and he wanted to do that. We waited until a few days before my flight to see if it would actually happen. I worked hard at keeping an open mind. If it worked, great! If it didn't, I would attend some concerts in San Francisco and find attention-grabbing local activities. I would be disappointed, but I could deal with it. Managing my anticipation and uncertainty was easier than dealing with Dave's.

A big factor here is that Alzheimer's patients do not do well with ambiguous situations. Because I had to wait until the last minute to know whether respite care would be available, it was hard to relay the information to Dave. I never could guess how far ahead of an event to inform him. Giving him the information too soon would mean repeated questions and concerns about what was going to happen. Springing information too close to the event was confusing to him and seemed cruel. In this case, I was preparing for a big trip and separation time. I didn't think it was a good idea to share the plan until close to departure.

I was happy and relieved when we learned for sure that the facility would have space for Dave and Dan during the appointed week. I hoped Dave would understand that he would be staying there for a week while I went to New York and that Dan would be there as well. Trying to promote a smooth transition, Joanie and I thought it would be good idea to double date for dinner at the facility the evening before the men moved in. We arranged to dine in the main dining room to make it easy for the guys to see the environment. While there, we could check out the scene and see how things worked. We made a reservation and pulled into the parking lot simultaneously.

The concierge ushered us to the private dining room rather than the main one. When we objected mildly, she said that Alan, the marketing director would join us shortly. We left a vacant chair for him at the head of the table. When our dinner was served, we assumed that he would join us soon. I saw Alan walk by in the hallway. He looked in on us with no sign of recognition, although Joanie and I had each had extensive meetings with him. That seemed rather strange, but I assumed he had other responsibilities and would join us shortly.

We finished dinner. I offered to see if I could find Alan. I did. He was in the reception area with a small monkey in the crook of his arm. Alan was bent over talking with a tiny nonagenarian in a wheelchair. The monkey looked bigger than the woman and somewhat threatening. When I approached Alan and introduced myself, he said, "I was expecting to find you in the main dining room and thought you had decided not to come."

Without missing a beat, he joined us in the private dining room. He was still toting the simian and told us way more about it and its habits and idiosyncrasies than we wanted to know. Since we thought this gathering was about the upcoming respite stay, we kept waiting for him to get to the point. That never happened.

Another part of the evening's agenda was for Joanie to finalize the contract for Dan's stay and sign some forms. Alan found Melanie, the executive director with whom Joanie had arranged a meeting. Melanie went to get the forms. She returned, saying that they were nowhere to be found and Joanie must not have turned them in. They had the forms from Dan's previous stay. Joanie's color heightened, but she maintained her composure. Melanie informed her that since they didn't have Dan's health data, he would need to get a TB test before he could stay. (It takes 4 days to evaluate the results of that test.) Joanie's color went up another notch. "Or, he could just get a chest X-ray," Melanie offered.

"Just" included taking an elderly man who adamantly objected to any kind of X-ray to a medical facility. He would have to wait (with no prior appointment) for up to half a day for the evaluation on the day he was to check into the assisted living facility.

Joanie and I glanced at each other. I could see the whole plan dissolving before my eyes. Melanie returned to her office and then invited Joanie in for a private conference. When Joanie emerged, she said, "We worked it out."

We left the building with our confused spouses at least an hour later than we had intended. We agreed that the visit hadn't accomplished our goal. It was one of my more bizarre experiences on the caregiving pathway and did nothing to inspire confidence that respite care, let alone assisted living could be a good idea. We followed through anyway. Dave's stay in respite while I went to New York went well. We talked every day on the phone. That was difficult because of his hearing issues, problems with phone access, and the need to be direct and concrete while talking about simple subjects. Despite those obstacles we made contact, and his morale was good.

Upon returning home after this week-long separation, a new care system was in place. Dave was attending LARC three days a week. After nearly three years in Walnut Creek, I was starting to establish a rhythm in my life that supported nourishing activities for me. Through a referral from someone in the Alzheimer's support network, a kind, competent, multi-talented caregiver, Antonio (Jun) Chan, found his way into our lives, and he spent every Friday with Dave allowing me to be away from home from 9:00 A.M. to 5:00 P.M.

Caregivers like Jun are worth their weight in gold and are not easy to find, but my weekly day of freedom came at significant financial cost: $200 per day. It was worth it! In addition to the financial cost of LARC, $70 per session, the 11:00 A.M. – 3:00 P.M. program schedule required that I leave home with Dave around 10:30 A.M., drop him off at 11:00 and then make the trip again at 2:30 P.M. It was approximately 2 hours driving for 3 hours respite. Timing was important. Dave could be a little late for the 11:00 A.M. session, but the 3:00 P.M. pick up had to be on time. All this left small opportunity for deep involvement in projects, outings or anything that required travel or concentration. This part became easier when I found a driver to take Dave to LARC, but that too cost money.

There was an invisible price tag that I would never have known about without direct experience. It's sort of like cleaning your house to prepare for the housecleaner. Jun and I would have a few minutes to talk before I left for the day, but if there were anything beyond the usual, I wrote things down. Here's a note I left for him on one occasion:

February 26, 2016

Medication management:

    In addition to bronchitis, Dave has a UTI. Dr. Fang added an antibiotic, LEVOFLAXIN that needs to start today.

    In addition to the antibiotic, Dave needs to take a probiotic, LACTINEX, 2 X a day. It's in the fridge.

    LEVOFLAXIN can be taken after lunch – but there can be no

milk products in the lunch. Sometime today, though, he should eat a
container of yogurt.
    Also, there is one more ZITHROMYCIN he needs to take.
Here's what I have in mind:
    Regular meds with breakfast, plus the ZITHROMYCIN.
    LACTINEX some time mid morning.
    LEVOFLAZIN after lunch (no milk products in lunch).
    Yogurt mid afternoon.
    Then, I will deal with evening meds and LACTINEX later.
I hope this makes sense. Call me if it's confusing.
    The beds need to be changed. And, if you would like to cook, we
have everything to make the chicken/artichoke casserole. Artichoke
hearts are in the freezer (TJ's in a bag.) If you would like to make
something else, that's great. I have magic rice that I can fix as
needed.
    Dave is actually feeling better than he has been. It's fine to go for
a walk or movie if you would like to do that. Please call if needed.
ENJOY THIS BEAUTIFUL DAY!

Yes, I could leave the house, but sometimes by the time I was out the
door, I felt like I had been through the wringer and had little energy left.

During Jun's initial interview, Dave, Jun and I had discussed some
of the challenges involved in caring for elderly people. He shared with
us that some of his patients had barely been able to communicate, but
Jun was able to maintain connection with them. I will never forget the
look of kindness and compassion on his face when he said, "They can
still say thank you."

Jun began coming to our house every Friday from 9:00 A.M. to 5:00
P.M., which allowed me to go to Qigong class in the morning, lunch and/
or a walk at noon, and an art class from 1:00 P.M. to 4:00 P.M. He and
Dave worked out a routine that Dave was happy about, including doing
laundry and cleaning house. I had discovered that Jun was a professional
cook. I didn't deprive him of the opportunity to make supper. His kindness,
intelligent talent, and compassion sustained Dave and me through a very
difficult year.

In November 6, 2017, I invited Jun to an interview about his work
as a caretaker and learned some things from his perspective. He had been

employed in the business about 13 years. He worked first as a caregiver and then as a house manager. He then began overseeing several facilities and trouble-shooting with management and staff before he moved into private care exclusively.

One of the things that had been difficult for me was telling Dave that I needed help and no longer felt comfortable leaving him home alone. I learned this is a common issue. I asked Jun for his wisdom about when it is time to get help. His answer was direct, "When you reach the time that caregiving is affecting your quality of life, you can't do what you want during the day, and you're not getting enough sleep. You could end up worse than the patient."

Some of Jun's suggestions for talking with the patient about introducing a caretaker and moving ahead with higher levels of care include:

- Never say a "caretaker" is coming. Use the term "companion," someone who will become your new friend and have interests like yours.

- Never say a companion is here to take over your care. The patient will still have his freedom of making decisions and choosing things that they like.

- No one will be telling you what is right or wrong. Your companion will be here to make sure you are safe and comfortable.

- In order to work effectively with a family, the caretaker needs the family to be open, make suggestions, and share information about the patient. That will aid the caretaker in building a relationship. It is essential to have a climate of mutual trust. "If I sense they cannot open up, I feel like they don't have trust. I can't bring good work. If they want me to do something that isn't fitting for the client, I need to speak up."

- When you feel like your home is turning into a hospital, it may be time to consider moving your loved one to assisted living. At this stage, it is important to find a place that is safe and well managed, where the level of activity matches that of the patient.

After our conversation, Jun sent me a follow-up email:

In thinking about our conversation, the most important thing I can say to the families who are thinking of getting in-home care is to look for caretakers who have compassion. Caretakers should be positive and able to uplift the patient's morale. Let them (loved ones) feel that they are still important. Give them a chance to tell what they need and ask what they think. Give them options, and they can choose for themselves. This will let them know that they still have a say. Let them feel that they are needed by the family and that will help make them feel important, not a burden. As I always say no matter how bad is their dementia, they will always have feelings. It's really rewarding when they give thanks in their own way and sometimes they will call your name until the end.
-Jun C.

When time for the Canadian music festival in August 2016 approached, I called the assisted living facility and did what I could to arrange for Dave to have another respite stay. It was the same procedure, including the interview with the nurse, a recent TB test and health data. They couldn't commit until just before time to fly. By now I was a bit inured to the process, and numbed by all I was dealing with. If it worked, it worked. If not…

They did have rooms for Dave and Dan.

Journal note: July 29, 2016
I dropped Dave off at the assisted living place on Thursday, July 28, 2016, for a ten-night stay. I felt incredibly sad. My chest hurt. This was unlike dropping him off before my New York trip in April. At that time I felt relieved and excited. I was surprised at my reaction and am still not clear about it. I thought I would feel happy and relieved. Instead I felt like crying and crying – but didn't. My best guess is that I am clearer about my profound loss, and it is closer to the time when Dave will go to assisted living. When I picked him up on my return, he was delighted to see me and to come home. I am going to have a very hard time with the next move.

Heartbreak Hill. I struggled for my own vitality and wanted the best for Dave. I knew I couldn't drag him, wounded, from the battlefield and save myself, too. A Qigong friend sent me this section from the poem "Bodhisattva Vows" by Albert Saijo.*

You're spending all
Your time and energy getting other people
Off the sinking ship into lifeboats bound
Gaily for Nirvana while there you are
Sinking, and of course you had to go and give
Your lifejacket away, so now let us be
Cheerful as we sink, our spirit ever
Buoyant as we sink.

Some good things were happening, though. Our care system was in place: LARC four days a week, and Jun on Fridays. Before being in this situation, I never would have had a glimmer about needing a driver. The trip to and from LARC was at least 40 minutes times 2, and it ended up being more like an hour each way. A HUGE gift from the support group was finding a paid driver. This basically added two hours of "free" time to each day Dave went to LARC, i.e. eight hours a week. Almost a whole workday!

There was a monthly price tag:
LARC - $1000.00
Jun - $ 800 to $1000.00
The driver - $400.00

Money is always an issue.

I had engaged enough help to construct a rickety vehicle of life that seemed good for Dave and allowed for my self-care, art and friends. My conveyance worked on an unpredictable schedule, which I crammed myself into as best I could. The carriage didn't always run on time, but it allowed me moments of grace.

CHAPTER 10

Assisted Living?
September 2016

I was caught between the overwhelming questions of WHEN and HOW to break the news to Dave. I had known for months that sometime soon, he needed to move to assisted living for his safety and wellbeing as well as for my sanity and physical health. Still, I couldn't bring myself to initiate the process. No time seemed like a good time. It was all just too awful.

Any family facing this decision has much to consider. Real and imagined dangers and challenges in the world of assisted living were concerns as I contemplated my own and Dave's personal issues regarding his placement. Besides needing to face the inevitable END, Alzheimer's patients and caregivers continue life in a complex, dynamic environment. Economic, environmental, and family needs and pressures influence opportunities and decisions. Bad stuff happens. Loss is a constant companion. We've all heard horrible tales of neglect and mistreatment of helpless elders. The expense of caretakers and/or assisted living is staggering.

But wait. There's more. People with dementia, just because of the age factor, are likely to have other serious medical conditions, and decisions about treatment are complex. In addition to Alzheimer's, Dave's aortic stenosis (his heart problem) was a major factor in pushing me toward a decision point. Beginning in April 2014, the family, including Dave, had been in discussion with a Kaiser team of cardiologists about the possibility of heart surgery to replace Dave's shrinking aortic valve. We had decided to decline the surgery.

On November 14, 2015, Dave awakened around 7:00 A.M. He had chest pains and was short of breath. He was sweating, very pale, and he was nauseous. I drove him to the Emergency Room, a mile and a half from our house. He was having a heart attack.

While he was in the hospital that evening, his palliative care doctor and I had a conversation with him that felt necessary but brutal. Understandably, Dave was frightened. The cardiologist had mentioned that it might be time to do the Transarterial Valve Replacement (TAVR) procedure. Dave was again considering that possibility. We tried, as kindly as possible, to explain to him that he had a progressive neurological disease that was ultimately going to make him unable to recognize us or care for even his most basic needs. The TAVR surgery, even though it wasn't open-heart surgery, would be very hard on him. I couldn't bring myself to say, "You could end up with a functional heart, but a brain that no longer allowed you to recognize or speak to us." Because I couldn't say those words, I don't think he understood clearly what the issues were.

The next day he was moved by ambulance from Walnut Creek Kaiser Hospital to San Francisco where a stent was placed in a blocked artery. Dave did well and was released the following afternoon. I was grateful that Karen drove us home from San Francisco.

We scheduled appointments with the San Francisco cardiac team after Thanksgiving. My sense was that Dave wanted the TAVR surgery. I couldn't see myself withholding it, even though I thought it was a very bad idea. I became resigned to the idea that surgery and all it implied was likely to be a next step.

Once again, Karen, Erica, Rex, Dave, and I met with the cardiac team and human resource people to consider the TAVR procedure. This time the approach was different from our previous TAVR exploration in Santa Clara. Dave went in for neurological testing. The surgical team met with Erica and Rex. The social worker met with Karen and me to discuss end-of-life decision issues. We divided up this way because Erica is a chiropractor, knowledgeable about the body, and Karen and I have psychological backgrounds. I felt that the momentum was toward Dave having the surgery and I was trying to keep my mind and heart open.

In our meeting with the social worker, Karen asked what experience she had had with dementia patients who underwent the TAVR procedure. Also, what was known about the effects of anesthesia on people with dementia? For the first time, I felt we received a clear answer about this, and I appreciated this woman's honesty. I didn't document her exact words, but she let us know these patients don't do well. Most never return to their previous level of cognitive functioning after the anesthesia, and the physical impact of the surgery is significant. Recovery is hard and slow. This is what I had gleaned from my informal research, but no one on either medical team had said it. The social worker also commented that there are wide variations on the level of care necessary after the TAVR has been performed.

Karen and I were finished with our meeting first. The person who had administered Dave's neurological evaluation came out to talk with us. She said, "You're going to have to explain something to me because I don't understand. Dave knows he is in San Francisco, why he is here, and he seems to understand what the surgery is. He doesn't know what day it is, has very little recall, poor judgment, and failed more than half of the exam I just gave him. I am trying to determine if my evaluation is valid or if I am way off base."

Karen and I looked at each other. This is what we had been dealing with over the past two or three years, at least. He could intermittently "pass." Dave appeared to be much more functional than he was. He could engage socially, and empathically, but he couldn't remember what happened a few minutes ago and couldn't follow an interaction. "Your evaluation is valid," we told her. "We see Dave in social situations where multiple conversations occur, and he passes as a fully-functioning, delightful older man. He covers his disability well."

Both the woman who had done the evaluation and I let our relief show. Her results were valid and my perceptions were affirmed. The way Dave appeared to strangers did not reveal his disability. She said she needed to talk with the surgical team. Over her shoulder she said something like, "When dealing with doctors, sometimes we need to beat them over the head with the non-medical stuff." I wanted to hug her.

While the social worker went off to meet with the doctors, our family, including Dave, had a big discussion. Our conversation was honest, direct and we laid out the painful truth. Dave had a serious heart condition. He had a progressive neurological disease. The choice was between surgery to address the heart issue, a risky prospect, or work to preserve his current quality of life between now and when either he had a fatal heart attack or faded into the oblivion of Alzheimer's. Dave spoke up and said he did not want the surgery. He would prefer for nature to take its course. Knowing him, he probably said, "her" course.

Each family member spoke in turn. Everyone concurred.

The surgical team knocked and entered our already cramped conference room. They seemed young, sincere, concerned and highly skilled. One of the doctors started to talk about the surgery. He looked like he wished he were having an Irish coffee on Union Street or anything that was far from where we were. I said, "Let me interrupt you. Dave and our family discussed the surgery thoroughly and decided that the TAVR is not a good idea for him. He has opted for a good quality of life for whatever time he has left." Dave chimed in and supported my assertion, as he had a thousand times in our work together.

I expected that we would receive the same response we had from the Santa Clara team, promoting the TAVR surgery. I was wrong. One of the young doctors smiled. "I'm honored to know your family. I think this is a wise decision, although a very difficult one. We support you 100% and want to help in any way we can."

We had ended another chapter and wouldn't be re-visiting the TAVR question.

Dave's recent heart attack made this decision-making process very real and painful. As a family, we were able to be present, share the responsibility, and embrace the next steps. Each of us stepped up in our own way and said what we had to say. I was proud of us. Trauma doesn't always bring family members close together. We had been in a crucible of life and death decision-making as a family and had found our way through it. I could see clearly that Dave's care needs had reached a point where I could no longer manage on my own.

Early on I was shocked to discover that caretakers at home, when I could find them, charged $20-30 per hour, with a five-hour minimum. I didn't feel like we could possibly afford that. As time passed, we began spending thousands of dollars a month for basic care, something that would have been beyond the realm of my imagination five years earlier.

"How could I justify spending money to avoid providing the care myself?" was one of the hardest questions I faced. My decision to place Dave in assisted living was aided by his inheritance, which he had received ten years earlier, a bright thread from his past. Without that available money, our options would have been fewer.

When a child is born, some families invest in that individual's advanced education. Not as many of us agree to sacrificing and saving for the inevitable expenses at life's end. When the question of insurance for long-term care came up when I was middle aged, I didn't even consider it seriously. I didn't want to confront the possibility that I might be a disabled elder, and for sure Dave couldn't. We needed our income for on-going expenses. I wasn't ready to acknowledge and prepare for death in a direct and conscious way. Many of us would rather our children inherit any resources we have been able to accumulate than lay out extraordinary amounts for end of life care. Denial owns lots of real estate.

In addition to the financial burden, many other factors determine whether or not placement will work. The decision becomes overwhelming. Although I have heard of a few cases, hardly anyone wakes up some morning and says, "I would really like to go to assisted living." People who are significantly beyond the limits of their home caregiver's capacity to care for them adamantly and violently, protest. Assisted living venues may not accommodate those who can't fit into the environment.

The mental and physical health of the prospective resident is a major factor in determining the success of placement. Will s/he have the capacity to embrace the move and thrive in the new environment after a reasonable period of adjustment? The terrible double bind here is that, for many complicated reasons, we wait until the patient has declined beyond having the ability to move into a strange environment to decide. One professional in the field had said to me that it is good to place people while they can still adjust to a new environment. I wasn't sure I believed it, but that made sense to me, and the idea supported me in making the decision.

Change is hard for all of us. For people with dementia, change is on a continuum from frightening to terrifying. Often one sees resistance, anger, and depression in dementia patients. These responses may become exaggerated due to limited capacity for emotional regulation when the individual is asked, or forced, to make a major life change. We cannot predict how a particular person will respond under these circumstances.

After it became clear to me that Dave was a candidate for assisted living, I did as much as I could to prepare him (and myself) for that move. I tried to think of what it would be like if I were the patient. Given his limited capacity to track and remember, I could only make my best guesses and proceed accordingly. During the summer of 2016, I hatched an idea that Dave could move after his 85th birthday in February, although, as I thought about it, I wondered if I could hold out that long.

On Friday, September 16, 2016, a friend from LARC's Alzheimer's support group, called me urging me to check out a brand-new assisted living complex that was opening that weekend. It was called Meadow and located in a nearby suburb. Most of the rooms had already been reserved, she said, and she was considering placing her mother there. This woman, a social worker who at that time sold hospice programs to a wide variety of facilities throughout the East Bay, was familiar with the facilities in this part of the world, and I trusted her judgment.

My friend's urgency upended me. Her recommendation was persuasive despite its unexpected intrusion on my current longer-term plan. I wasn't ready to act, and my automatic resistance flared: Meadow was too expensive, too fine, and too impossible. Several friends had asked me, "Why wait?" Although I could spin plausible reasons, my answers were consistently unclear. Denial slowed my thinking. It was too hard to believe that Dave really needed to move. As I hashed and rehashed the phone call, I had the same feeling I had when we listed the house for sale. Was this really happening? I felt like I had just overturned a snow globe, was waiting for the flakes to fall, and the whole scene was in another universe.

The move had to happen. No time was the right time. I decided to see what I could learn. That night my mind went to a decision-making carnival rather than messing around with something as mundane and necessary as sleep. The Ferris wheel circled round and round, offering different perspectives from each elevation, shifting from one view to another with frightening speed. The scene altered with each turn.

On Friday, before I received the call about Meadow, I'd had a brief conversation with Jun, Dave's kind and experienced care person, as I was heading out for my day's activities. We didn't have much time for discussion, but in passing I mentioned that I thought it might be time for Dave to go to assisted living. To my surprise, Jun agreed that Dave would be better off in assisted living than at home, and that it was time to make the move. We didn't get to explore in depth, but his comment stayed with me. Why hadn't I consulted him before this?

Dave and Dan, the friend he had met at LARC, his respite program, had gone to weeklong respite stays at another facility twice during the previous April and August, and had done well. Dan's wife, Joanie, and I had discussed *ad nauseam* assorted strategies for placing the men in the same facility with the thought that they could be support for each other.

Respite is one experience, residence another. A time-limited stay at an assisted living facility is much less daunting than moving in for the rest of your life.

Joanie, along with two family members, our social worker friend, Karen, Spencer, and I went to check out Meadow, despite my initial resistance. Since no residents had yet moved in we were able to look at all the spaces in both assisted living and in the memory care unit. By then, Karen and I had explored at least six other communities of this type and had bases for comparison. Meadow was brand-new, a beautiful facility with 83 total spaces, 30 of which were in memory care.

On our visit to Meadow that day, we had too many people for our interview and too little time. The regional director for the Meadow organization was game for embracing the task, though, and acted as if this were the usual way things were done. She answered our questions, guided us around, and pointed out features of the environment. We paid the totally refundable deposit and signed the men up to become some of the first residents in this complex.

After signing we had 45 days to move in. I was thinking around early November would be a good time, but wanted to coordinate with Joanie to arrange for Dave and Dan to move in about the same time. I knew that Meadow was having an open house the following week, and my plan was to talk with Dave about the move and then take him to the open house. I wanted to be sure the plan was in place before engaging him.

That week was exceptionally busy. As I floated through this time, I was completely absorbed with decision-making and thinking about how I could have the inevitable talk with Dave about his move to assisted living. This decision was as life-changing as the move from Sacramento. I didn't want to open the discussion too far ahead of time because it would elevate Dave's anxiety, and he would have questions, understandably, that would be repeated many times because of his inability to remember the answers. With the open house looming on Saturday, though, I had to find space and time for a sit down.

I had dedicated energy and thought to creating an honest, supportive, clean, and effective approach for carrying our process forward. I had asked for input from family, friends, and whomever I thought could help me. I had made notes. The main ideas focused on my no longer being able to provide for Dave's care, that doing so was affecting my health, and that I needed his help in dealing with the next stages of our lives. I would also focus on the importance of his safety and wellbeing.

Mini-rehearsals for THE TALK skittered through my thoughts, chained around me, seeped into my pores, owned me. I could think of little else and moved through time with friends who were visiting in a trance. I was glad they were with me offering support and distraction. By Thursday, I knew I needed to have THE TALK but didn't have a good time to do it until after Dave, our visitor and I watched a baseball game and went to bed about 10:00. P. M. I was afraid Dave would be too tired to think, not to mention the chaos in my own thoughts.

When it occurred to me to begin the talk the way many talks in the past had begun, I felt a little hope. I was as prepared as I could be, and the only thing to do was to go for it. "We have come to a place in our lives where we need to make some big decisions that neither one of us wants to face…" I started.

I described Meadow to Dave and shared how I had discovered it. I let him know that Karen and I had been looking at assisted living facilities for some time and of all we had seen, this one seemed the best. I told him I felt sad about having to face this decision and knew he would also, but that it was inevitable. I asked him if he had seen it coming, and he said no. I talked about feeling stressed and that I worried about his well-being. He said he knew that.

Finally, I decided to tell him what I had discovered on my week in Canada during the summer. "When I was away from home at the music festival last summer, I didn't feel pressure in my chest and the pains that I had been having."

He said he knew that I was stressed and tired and he didn't want that for me. "You are the most important thing in my life, and I don't want to be a burden. I have said that repeatedly."

"I know," I responded. "I know you want to do the right thing, and this is hard for you."

This conversation went on for a while - repeating and clarifying. It was like many conversations we had had over the years, and it felt like the "old Dave" was back. He showed the same empathy, kindness, love, and concern I have known throughout our years together, the reasons I loved him from the beginning. I believed him. This felt different from the other times he had said that if he needed to be "someplace else," I should make arrangements for that to happen. This conversation felt genuine, like he truly understood that we were both in a painful situation.

Dave had fallen two weeks earlier, and that had frightened him more than I realized. I was already making plans for the move, but his fall confirmed my judgment that the time was upon us. He agreed.

Sporadically, my mind became an adversary, trying to take me off track. I found myself feeling that his support and understanding of the whole process made it harder rather than easing my confusion. What was I thinking? How could I not continue to care for him at home? With effort, I pushed these thoughts away and didn't voice them to Dave.

I thought about the fall, the repeated questions, his disorientation to time and space, his mixing up our friends and not remembering who lives in Santa Fe, who in Santa Barbara. I felt like it was the best decision I could make in a no-win situation. That night I slept better than I had for weeks. I was sad but relieved.

At some point when I was researching feminine mythology for a workshop I was doing, I encountered a story about Persephone, sometimes known as Queen of the Underworld, and how, during her journeys between the upper and lower worlds, she encountered horrifying dangers. Her mother, Demeter, provided her with loaves of bread, which she had to guard and preserve. At just the right moment, she could toss the bread to the vicious monsters who guarded the passage to and from the underworld. She could thus distract them, enabling her to slip through unharmed. In guarding her loaves, she had to say no and to protect her resources from many in dire circumstances who begged and pleaded for food. Her temptations toward self-sacrifice were overwhelming at times, but she held on. I remember the story, although I can't find the reference, and it fueled my determination to preserve myself. Countless times, though, I felt like it would be simpler to throw the loaves to the desperate ones and collapse into caregiving forever.

Monday following THE TALK we made a list of things Dave would like to take with him to his new place. My goal was to begin grounding our plans and make them real. He participated. The family was 100% supportive. They let me know that they understood, and asked what they could do to help. Although I knew this was just the initiation of the move and the physical and logistical work were ahead for me, I had direction and felt deep relief.

But I wasn't going to get off easy. On Friday evening, less than 24 hours after THE TALK, an acquaintance stopped by for an impromptu visit. She was someone I had met whom I thought might be a good walking buddy and friend.

I wanted to tell somebody that we had decided that Dave would go to Meadow just to see how it would feel to share this information. Since the process had developed quickly, I hadn't told anyone outside family and very close friends that we were thinking in that direction, although I wasn't exactly keeping it a secret. I don't know what I expected, but I sure didn't expect what happened. She let me know that I was making a mistake, that it was a terrible decision, that I was being foolish, which she later amended to shortsighted. Her opinion was that I was seduced by the glitz of a new facility and that I was thinking more of myself than of Dave.

Through my haze, I was able to say, "Wait a minute! I am super vulnerable right now. I don't need for you to agree, but take it easy!"

She said, "I'm sorry if you're vulnerable, but I have to say what I really believe. I think that place is way too big for someone like Dave. He will get lost there, and it's too far from where you live to drive as much as you're going to need to." She explained some more of her objections, not that she needed to. She had just targeted my worst fears and activated them.

At that point I was glad that I had had experience as the object of pointed disagreement. I realized I was attempting to justify my decision, and stopped. I was able to say: I think the best thing we can do is agree to disagree. She walked off shaking her head. I was shaking all over.

The next morning Dave and I met Karen and her family at Meadow for the open house. We found the parking lot jammed, with valets parking newcomers. A pianist held forth on the grand piano in the living room. Noise, crowd, chaos. Dave looked overwhelmed and confused. Several times he repeated to staff people that he had been there before. They smiled, nodded, and went on to the next thing.

We were able to see the apartment that I had reserved for Dave. He looked around it and said, "This is a nice-sized room," and sounded sincere. I was relieved. It was a studio with adequate space but just enough room for his bed, recliner, TV, and a few occasional pieces. The private bathroom had a good shower with grab bars and a bench. The room featured an outside window and a decent street view. I could furnish the space in a way that would feel welcoming and comfortable.

Dave and I had a constructive follow-up talk after dinner at home. I no longer felt like a bad person who was stowing her partner away. I felt like a responsible person doing a hard thing. Dave's part-time caregiver, Jun, and his son would come to move Dave's furniture on Sunday. Dave's first night there would be the following Wednesday, October 12, 2016, leaving him just three more nights in our home. I trusted some relief would happen after the move. It seemed like each step was heavy. That morning at Qigong, as our practice group meditated, I felt deep sadness. I was more in touch with loss than relief, and I knew the loss had been creeping forward for years.

Dave had been thinking that if Meadow didn't work out, he would come back to living with me. I had tried to clarify that would not be the case, that if Meadow didn't work out, he would be going to another assisted living facility. I was glad he had LARC early the next week as a distraction, giving me time to finish wrapping up details for the move. It seemed both simple and overwhelming. On one hand there was not that much to move, and yet I was facing the biggest challenge of my life in the direction of decline. Dave's move to assisted living was an acknowledgement that Alzheimer's was in command. We could no longer maintain the fantasy that we controlled our direction, if not our destiny.

Having THE TALK ranks high in the hardest things I have ever done in my life, and I knew there were more hard steps coming. It was a great gift to me that Dave was still able to be supportive and that he comprehended this was something we needed to do. I had no expectation that he would be able, or willing, to move over in that direction, but when he did, it was consistent with the way he had been throughout our relationship.

I was relieved. I could almost imagine being happy and light-hearted again, but it was too early to lower my guard. The decision had been made, but the move was yet to come.

A period of adjustment loomed ahead.

CHAPTER 11

Dave's Move
September and October 2016

Wheels of change crunched on after the decision was in place. Three busy weeks buffered the time between the decision and the move. Two friends and Judy came to spend time with us. Judy and I went to Winslow, Arizona, for my 60th high school reunion, and Dave and I took a long-awaited road trip to Santa Barbara to visit friends. These distractions helped in some ways, padding the time with nourishing activity. Judy and friends were aware of our situation and helped by talking with us about the layers of change we faced and the challenges of aging, as well as comforting us with good food, music, and loving company.

Concurrently, I arranged for the move, which involved two main features: 1) Dave and his personal items, and 2) the furniture and supplies to make his new apartment homey and comfortable. My first thought was that the whole move would happen in one day. I came to my senses in time to contract with Jun and his son to help us with the furniture a few days before Dave's personal move-in date.

I thought it would be sad for Dave to see his bed and belongings moved out of our house. It was sad for me. I created a strategy to soften the extraction. I asked the men in our family, Rex, Spencer, and his dad, to take Dave out to brunch on the Sunday morning before move-in while Jun and his son transported Dave's big furniture items to Meadow. Erica, Karen and I followed the movers and arranged the details in Dave's apartment, made the bed, and then Erica and Karen virtually held my hand while I dithered. Jun had to make two trips in his truck, taking longer than we anticipated. Our plan to have Dave away from home while we moved his things didn't work perfectly, but it worked well enough.

In the afternoon, Erica, Rex, and I took Dave to Meadow to see the space and tell us where he would like to hang the paintings he had chosen. He looked around and said, "This is a nice-sized room," just as he had said when he had seen it during the open house a few weeks earlier. I felt relieved and had a sense that this transition might be OK.

After getting through the furniture move on Sunday, my stress index dipped a bit but began climbing again on Monday. Time crawled. Minutes seemed like hours. I vacillated between the poles of feeling I was making a life-saving decision for myself that was right and necessary on one hand and that I was a terrible person leading an innocent lamb to slaughter on the other. I had yet to understand that Dave would actually be better off in assisted living than he could be living at home.

Not only was this move emotionally laden, it had huge financial implications. Was I capable of such responsibility? If not me, who? Once again I appreciated why people continue to soldier on toward total self-defeat rather than making a change. As I tried to sleep that night, I thought I might explode. Sleep was not my friend. I used all my tricks, trying to relax to no avail, as I lay stiff and agitated in bed. I got up from time to time to pace and stretch.

October 12, 2016, Dave went to LARC and I drove to Meadow to be there as required for his TV installation, to give his room the final touches, and to make sure he had everything he needed. I hadn't showered. My hair was a mess, and I felt like I was approaching 100 years of age. My plan was to fluff and buff before picking him up at LARC at 3:00 P.M. and then to take him to Meadow where I would stay for dinner with him.

As I was leaving Meadow after the TV installation, trudging through the lobby with arms full of empty bags and packing paraphernalia, feeling like a gelatinous blob, I encountered the facility's executive director in her trim business suit and high heels. She greeted me in a friendly way and asked how things were going. She also said something kind with sincerity in her tone and put her hand on my shoulder. To my total surprise, I burst into tears, undignified snot slithering from my nose, salt water dripping off my chin. I struggled to manage some kind of recovery. Tactfully, this kind woman stepped into her office and grabbed some tissues for me, while I set my burden down and pulled myself together.

We talked briefly and she checked to see if I was OK to drive home.

I made that short trip in a daze, quickly showered, and continued to Orinda to pick Dave up at LARC for the move. He was in good spirits, and we both maintained well during the half hour drive to his new home.

As we drove up to Meadow, he said, "Is this my new home?"

"Yes, it is," I said in what I hoped was a good voice.

"But it doesn't mean we're getting a divorce?" he asked.

"Of course not," I managed.

We checked in, picked up his key and his care call medallion, which the concierge explained to him, and headed for his new home. We had dinner in the beautiful but mostly empty dining room. It was painful to see Dave accepting the reality that we were going to be separated. He said he felt sad. We talked about it again, several times, repeating that I could no longer take care of him and that I worried about him constantly. He still seemed to comprehend, and he acknowledged that he knew caring for him was taking a toll on me.

I can't remember the drive home that night other than I felt more leaden than light and was dead tired. Even though I had been working hard to gain relief, and my efforts had come to fruition, I couldn't feel any benefit. I was numb. Dave's courage and openness eased the transition in one way and were heartbreaking in others. He was disoriented, as expected, but I was disoriented too. I felt off balance and unsure of myself.

Journal entry October 15, 2016, Three days after the move

I feel like I have climbed into a Salvador Dali painting. The clocks are melting and the world is warped. I have spent hours – three, I think – getting my simple little TV set up because I took the big VIZIO to Dave's room at assisted living. I need assisted living – a full time TV tech consultant and gourmet meals served to me when I'm hungry – and now his TV, which I spent mucho attentianado making right - isn't working. I could scream, except that I'm too worn down and flat to exert that much energy. I can't believe it.

And, I do believe it. He probably hit the wrong button on the remote and now all he can get is Russian programming. I know it's no big deal. I just have to sort it out. It was just another annoyance, but extra layers of frustration keep appearing where I can't predict them, don't want them, and don't like them. I feel hope and I feel numb. I am really, really sick of it all and just want to go some place peaceful, beautiful and quiet and know that the thousands of dollars a month we are spending ensure that Dave is comfortable, secure and content. Can I buy peace?

I don't know what the roll out is going to be. I feel like I'm in the grasp of a monster and have lost any sense of control. It's not about being a person in the world trying to find my own way. It's about responsibility for the life of another human being who can't take care of himself and who doesn't have the wherewithal to initiate plans or know that our duplex rent is $3000 a month, not $300 which I overheard him say to someone a couple days ago.

By the next week I was in better shape, more centered and rested. Dave's move had been accomplished, and I was no longer on duty 24/7. My dreams continued with strange, confused imagery, and lack of control appeared prominently. Even though Dave was not living with me, I was tethered to his schedule. My days converged around transporting him to LARC and other places as well as visiting him at Meadow. I experienced a warp between relief from the moment-to-moment care pressure and the reality of my time centering on Dave's clock.

Dave seemed to be adjusting to his new environment, learning his way around and making the best of the situation. I admired his willingness to move into a life style that was not of his design or desire and do what he could to make it work. I hope I can be as brave when my turn comes. As I look back on this time, it is clear that moving him to Meadow while he had the capacity to make this adjustment was good strategy, not just a rationalization to make my life easier. As time went on and he became more confused and disoriented, it would have been much more difficult for him to move.

Through regular meetings with the care staff at Meadow, I was able to track Dave's health and adjustment in the new environment. In addition to formal assessments, they provided me with informal feedback from time to time. When I arrived unannounced, they welcomed me graciously by name and treated me as an honored guest. Servers in the dining room soon knew Dave's food and beverage preferences and brought them to him before he asked.

My life at home improved exponentially. I began playing my piano and vibraphone, something I hadn't felt like doing for ages. With regularity, I woke up by 7:00 A. M. and by 8:00. I was out for my walk, which included solo Qigong practice in the park. I felt my way along, shedding layers of protective numbness, enjoying moments of excitement as I honored my needs and interests rather than

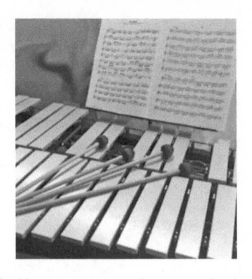

my projection of Dave's needs. I had been caregiving so long it was hard to imagine being free of the load, focused on my own perception of the world and my place in it.

And here is where we came to the deal I had made with the devil. LARC. Lamorinda Adult Respite Center had been a lifesaver for me and for Dave. The beautifully designed and executed program had been perfect for him. Although I didn't quite get the significance at the time, his seamless slide into that program had revealed the level of his impairment. Consequently, other than me, LARC had become the center of his life. The people there loved him and took wonderful care of him. He had made friends there, especially Dan, who had also moved into Meadow.

The first question Dave had asked about the move was whether he would be able to continue at LARC. Despite the expense, I felt that it would be cruel to have him leave the program. I accepted the fact that providing transportation back and forth three days a week (80 miles of driving each of those days) would keep me tied to Dave's schedule until he could truly connect with the program at Meadow.

Erica and Rex paid their first visit to Dave at Meadow and then stopped by to see me on their way back to their home in Santa Cruz. They thought Dave was in a better place emotionally than the last time they had seen him at home, and they liked Meadow. High praise considering their earlier opinion that placement in assisted living would be a bad idea. They had been supportive to me throughout the decision-making process, but now I felt palpable relief to have them truly on board with the decision.

I knew I couldn't have kept going as I was, but now I felt guilty, just like people in the Alzheimer's support group said I would. I wanted to move around in my life, write my book, and go where I wanted to go, when I wanted to go, without hurting Dave. I didn't want to watch him fall off the cliff and then not be able to find him as happened in a dream I had recorded recently. Throughout this period, friends expressed their care and concern and contacted me more frequently than usual. This support helped.

In a way, I knew this would happen: the taste of freedom made it that much more difficult to be tied to a schedule. What I needed to do was embrace the freedom I had and not dread filling my obligations. I thought I could do that. It would help to have a schedule of sorts that Dave could depend on and I could depend on. Predictability might make us both less anxious and me less resentful.

I was grateful that I felt more rested and less stressed. I wanted to embrace my freedom to get up and go for a walk, plan my day and have access to moving around in my own space at home. I wanted to flow with taking care of Dave and move from under *The Clamp*. He had been a good partner, loyal and true, and my job now was to manage his care in absentia while I enjoyed my life as much as possible.

After Dave had been at Meadow about a month, I took a long weekend trip to Santa Fe, solo, to visit my old friends Melissa and Jim. Traveling alone and being with our dear friends in a place where Dave and I had frequently visited felt strange, free and sad simultaneously. All I had to do was arrive at the airport, line up in the right place, and board the plane, much simpler than traveling with Dave. Jim picked me up at the Albuquerque airport, and then I was shortly in the beautiful space of their home, having dinner at a table for three. Bittersweet.

A month after Dave's move I made these notes about how different I felt and what I needed to sustain a healthy, creative life:

- I will make sure that Dave is well cared for, which doesn't mean I need to provide that care myself by living with him. I need more clarity about what it does mean, and I hope to find a rhythm that feels mutually supportive.
- I have the option to watch programs on TV that I choose and record things for later viewing. The schedule is no longer filled with sports.

- I have some schedule concerns, but they are fewer by far. Moving around in the world doesn't revolve on Dave's schedule 24/7 or on an hourly basis. I can get up in the morning, walk out the door to exercise and take as long as it takes.
- I'm having fun rearranging the house, making it fit my patterns and needs. I have never lived alone, and for now, at least, I am enjoying the buoyancy and freedom of a new life style.
- I'm excited about my new art room. It feels good to be in there working again.
- I look forward to taking small trips, including a few to Sacramento to see friends.
- I anticipate going to the symphony and to art events without having to make complicated arrangements. It was good to be in Santa Fe and to make the trip easily. Since Dave was at Meadow, I didn't have to plan and think through all the steps outside caretakers would need to provide for him.
- I can get up any time I wish, in the middle of the night, or sleep in, without organizing around caregiving.
- I can practice music on my own schedule, not timed around Dave's needs for rest or other requirements. It's hard to give myself permission. I still resist picking up my mallets or sitting down at the piano. I want to change that.
- I will continue to dismantle *The Clamp*, which still bears down, but not with its earlier weight.

Dave was doing all he could to embrace his new life and was getting along better than expected. With my freshly minted appreciation for every day, I looked forward to a walk on the trail, Qigong in the park, and lunch with a friend. Caregiving continued as part of the mix, but in a very different way. The time with Dave nested in a relatively predictable schedule, which included time away from caregiving.

I could breathe.

CHAPTER 12

Focus on Self-Care

"My husband has Alzheimer's," I say to a friend or to a new acquaintance. Their first response is invariably, "I'm so sorry!" Then they ask, "Does he still recognize you?" I say, "Yes." One common response to that is, "What a horrible disease!" There is a good possibility that they will add, "My mother (uncle, friend's father) has (had) Alzheimer's, and…" Then, finally, this polite and jarring conversation ends with, "*You really need to take care of yourself.*"

They intend genuine care and concern, and I plead guilty to having offered similar comments to others. Now, I shudder to recall my naiveté. Until I engaged in this late-life caregiver process, I had no clue what it felt like to be on the receiving end of, "*Take care of yourself.*" It is as if they are asking me to do something that is impossible. Every moment hasn't been hands-on caregiving, but every decision contained the element of Dave-care. When innocent people say, "*Take care of yourself,*" to me, I work hard to inhibit a dismissive response and to reassure them that their concern is appreciated. The terrible truth is that the whole situation is painful and complex, and you CAN'T take good enough care of yourself.

My mind feels like a kaleidoscope when I'm on the receiving end of well-intentioned comments that include, "…someone else in my family has (had) Alzheimer's," and "You need to take care of yourself." Too many thoughts want to be heard.

Watching your life partner fade into dementia, seeing his eyes glaze over, his athletic grace shift to a halting gait, and his once brilliant mind in chronic confusion is different from experiencing similar changes with anyone else. I'm not denigrating anyone's loss. I'm just saying that losing your life partner is different from other losses.

Research says that 12% of caregivers tend to a spouse or partner. And these aren't all dementia-related. "Women caregivers, as a group, have been found over and over to fare worse than men – and wives worst of all," *Scientific American Mind**. I have to say that when I read this horrible statistic I felt better because it affirmed my experience and made me feel less crazy.

After I realized that Dave was ill, not just being irresponsible or self-centered, one of my main feelings was that I ought to be able to do this caregiver thing better. He had been the love of my life, a wonderful partner both at home and at work, and a generous life companion. It's hard to remember, but he was also sexy and fun. Much of the literature about caregiving describes spiritual growth through providing excellent care for a loved one. Descriptions of caregiving are filled with stories about precious moments, humorous events, feelings of mastery and satisfaction in creating a safe, loving environment for the failing partner.

I would love to tell you that I found meaning in all these ways and embraced my job of caregiving every day. Unfortunately I can't. My story didn't fit the mold, which, in the early days, especially, contributed to deep feelings that I should be able to do this better. Of course I would take care of my partner, but I was also in a fight for my own healthy survival.

Self-maintenance is what I needed to do to stay alive and healthy. It is something I hadn't considered much in the past; it simply hadn't required close attention. As my caregiver responsibility increased, and I became aware that my stress level was rising, I could no longer stay on autopilot and maintain my current life style. I needed to actively engage taking care of myself. It never occurred to me that such a process would require a significant portion of every single day. Although my basic care structure has remained the same over time, here is how it looked when Dave was still living at home:

- Journaling, including life events, dreams and insights
- Walking two miles every day
- Practicing Qigong (QQ) a traditional movement, meditation form, 20-40 minutes daily

Other self-maintenance activities included occasional facials or massages, going to the dentist, getting my hair done, and shopping for necessities like socks or linens. Any medical issues that needed attention fit here as well. All these things required both scheduling the event and Dave-care, and they invariably took longer than I thought they would. Each item that decorated the calendar reduced possibility of flexibility and spontaneity.

Self-nourishment had to do with mental/emotional health and a sense of well-being. How could I create the optimal amount of time and space for myself? My solitude could wear many different faces: contemplation, peace, sadness, freedom, the emptiness of wishing for contact, or even joy, and it was important to me.

Defining the separate categories of *self-maintenance* and *self-nourishment* clarified the self-care process, and it became more functional for me. Understanding that these facets were equally important was a challenging but necessary step for survival. I had a much more difficult time making *nourishment* a priority because it felt indulgent. It's not. I have learned that taking time out to do things we enjoy has big payoff in energy and sustenance when times are hard.

Maintaining the living environment, the *household* and all that involved could be a full-time job for any able-bodied person. In our family, Dave had taken more than his share of responsibility in this realm from the beginning of our relationship. However, when deciding which recycle "bucket" was the right one for each piece of trash became a major issue, and we had to discuss the reasons for each choice at length, I knew I could no longer rely on his help. His obsessiveness was overwhelming me and wearing me down. The garbage disposal ran for longer periods; the vacuum cleaner went on forever. Emptying the dishwasher generated more questions than I could field. Self-care began to include increasing my share of household management, car maintenance, bill paying, and all relevant correspondence while maintaining the fiction that Dave was still doing most of it.

What happens when a person can no longer carry on their daily lives doing the things that have made them feel like themselves? What is left? Dave had been a well-respected psychologist in a university setting and in private practice. He was socially active and lovingly involved with his family. He could no longer load the dishwasher without help or carry on a conversation. How could that feel?

When Jun began helping us, he made a major contribution to housecleaning and was able to include Dave in the process. He knew how to support Dave. That was a sea change for me, relieving stress I didn't know I had.

Caregiving was not made easier by the fact that Dave and I left Sacramento just when his illness was becoming critical. We had spent more than four decades in that community weaving networks of friends, colleagues and acquaintances and knew only two people in Walnut Creek other than Karen and her family. Building a support network in our new environment became a priority for me. The way I knew to go about this was to take classes at the community center, local studios or other resources in subjects that interested me. My first try was a photography class where only three other people showed up. One dropped out. I finished the class and enjoyed it immensely. It was a modest start in getting out and about, but it wasn't a successful social venture. Later attempts in Qigong and art classes were rich in connecting me with people who became friends.

Our immediate *family* plus my sister Judy and Dave's sister Nora have all helped in countless ways with both hands-on assistance and moral support. Cousin Carolyn's wisdom held me. They have been there for the hard decisions and have supported us as we have taken each step in this uncharted, perilous journey. Asking for their help and accepting it began a new chapter in my life. Spending time, including email, FaceTime and phone conversations, with *friends,* both old and new, has been a cornerstone of self-care for me. Several of my old best friends from Sacramento have come to visit from time to time, to share an adventure in the city or in some other part of the magnificent Bay Area. Since mobility has been hard for me, these gifts were even more meaningful.

Experience and research tell us about the vulnerability of caregivers. Many get sick and die before the object of care departs. Others are long-suffering, self-denying and make it through to the other side. Another group finds meaning in caregiving, embracing the process and continuing to provide care to others when their loved ones pass. Just like dementia affects people differently, taking care of oneself as a caregiver looks different to all of us. "*Take care of yourself*" is excellent advice though its many layers slip and slide even while under construction.

For me, and for others I know in this caregiver situation, the self-care conversation nearly always circles through "What is self-care, and what is self-indulgence?" For most of us, it is challenging to embrace the practice of self-care because, in the face of our loved one's illness it feels indulgently self-centered! I've thought about this from many different angles, and it is easy to see how and why other people, rather than myself, need to take self-care seriously. It took having fatigue and chest pains for me to legitimize my own needs enough to change my lifestyle.

What I have learned about self-care. Hard as it has been to commit, I look at my calendar BEFORE I schedule something or agree to be some place or do something with or for someone. My body can no longer accomplish my mind's yearnings or perceived obligations. After I realized that I was over-reacting to canceled plans and other abrupt disappointments, I took on the job of getting better at handling these situations. Sometimes I choose to say NO to things I would really LIKE to do and trust another enjoyable opportunity will emerge.

My friends and acquaintances who are members of our special unintended caregiver network agree that no one can know what it is like to be in this situation unless they are members too. Can anyone judge the way I manage it? No, nor should I judge myself (or others) by my old standards.

Each of us needs to create some kind of personal support system for self-care through this time of stress. Here's a list of how I endeavor to be mindful and maintain a here-and-now orientation and some degree of flexibility. This is just my list, not necessarily relevant for anyone else. It takes energy and discipline to stay on track, and sometimes it is harder to stay consistently involved with this list than others.

- Maintain Qigong practice even when inconvenient, I don't have time, or I feel too tired.
- Go for my walk, rain or shine.
- Write in my journal and do my dream work, even when I can barely remember the dream or I don't have time, as well as when clarity hits.
- Stay tuned to patience and compassion as self-care, not sainthood.
- Focus. Attend to the here and now. Relinquish journeys into the past.
- Practice self-nourishing ways rather than feeling undeserving.
- Honor past relationships and present ones as well.
- Practice music an hour a day.
- Do at least one fun (frivolous) thing every day, as simple as a half hour reading *The New Yorker*. Reserve room for more than that.
- Think about what else should be on this list.

OK. This list is idealistic, but I've found over time, that I can do much of it. And, when I can stick to it, the world may go to hell around me, but I feel more energized and relaxed than when I skip it or can't do it.

In addition to my life's unpredictability, another disruption glowers at me. My energy pool has limits. Taking care of two people requires at least twice as much fuel as taking care of one person. If tired, I rest or take a nap and try to resist the temptation to push through drowsiness or fatigue. My body is talking about my needs for regeneration. Self-care can be more boring than stimulating because it seems like spending a lot of time on maintenance. Going for a walk isn't always interesting, and practicing music requires more energy than sitting on the couch, but I feel better when I follow through than when I collapse. Sometimes I try to use boredom as meditation, part of learning to relax rather than spinning my wheels with impatience. I rarely succeed. I'm a work in progress.

For a while I experimented with acting as if I were pregnant and allowed myself permission to be careful with my energy. I got over the need for that ruse. Now I feel free to change plans I have made with others if effort outweighs reward, or if I just can't want to do it. I'm not pregnant, but I am more delicate than I used to be and deserve to protect my energy. I am not as important as I sometimes think and don't have to overextend myself just because I said I would be there!

At a more subtle level I pay attention if I feel anxious or depressed rather than going on to the next thing. Those discomforts are alerting me. I can dissolve my ROBOWOMAN denial and delve into taking whatever steps I need to do. I work to stay mindful and to prioritize.

My head doesn't feel as scrambled as it had for a long time. I decide the night before which project I want to work on and prepare for that. I select small bits in case I don't have the energy to tackle the whole thing. I try not to commit (even to myself) to projects I can't manage, and I do my best to keep my expectations small. It helps if I can clear off my workspace and enjoy a beautiful surround, but I can also sit in the middle of a mess and make tracks.

Being explicit about *taking care of myself* reminds me how much is involved. When Dave faded into dementia, a huge part of my life's nourishment went with him. Our romantic relationship stuttered and halted. Decades had flown since my boudoir harbored action. Nor did everyday life contain gentle nudges, flirting, feeling sexy, looking forward to my little black dress hitting the floor. Long ago, a once enjoyable sex life dwindled to non-existence. It is hard to remember. We talked about our loss and loneliness early on, attributing change to aging in general, and then the conversation evaporated.

The most private facet of our lives is not much acknowledged as part of the Alzheimer's story among the people I know. Even if I were able and willing to reveal my own intimate concerns, (don't worry, I'm not!) sharing Dave's side of the issue would be unacceptable.

Through the Alzheimer's Association and other sources available on line, some information about aging and sexuality is available for both the person with Alzheimer's and the caregiver. It is helpful and covers sexual activity in assisted living and how to manage relevant hygiene. It doesn't, and can't, deal with the moral and emotional aspects of the topic. For me, this is a knot I haven't untied. What if I happened upon someone I found especially attractive and interesting and the feeling was mutual?

Partly because of a long, satisfying relationship with Dave my feelings about loss of intimacy were overridden by my motivation to manage the logistical challenges we faced. I retreated into my favorite childhood defenses. Numbness and compartmentalization* served me well in shelving the reality of my sexuality.

Love, shared values and interests, compassion for the other, the big things that tether a relationship are familiar, but I had never considered the importance of whispers, a shared look, or a joke based on some long-past happening. Often these bits are sexual innuendos or intimations, tendrils of subterranean energy that will surface when the time is right. Dementia eradicated any semblance of subtlety, including old habits of non-verbal communication. This whole layer of connection disappeared.

Loss of the give and take of affection, a big part of self-care is the real subject here. Gray Panthers no doubt romp in the jungle, but for most of us sexual activity becomes a less prominent dimension of our lives as we age. We learn to accept this decline. We express and receive affection in conversation, good meals, shared events, travel, music and art, or other interests. Sexual distancing is one more loss of connection, increasing feelings of emptiness and vulnerability. Physical closeness and intimacy may have been the last part of our relationship to diminish. Intellectual sharing left first; and then emotional communication became direct and concrete, absent of nuance and understanding. I felt distanced and dispassionate.

Attraction is more than physical for me, and probably for most women who opt for long-term relationships. It has to do with trust, safety, willingness to be vulnerable, and desire to be understood. With diminished energy exchange in our relationship I felt objectified, like I was a thing.

Despite moving through life in this bland state, my unconscious, not easily silenced, was sending me messages through the dream channel.

Journal entry: September 16, 2010
Dream:

I am at a conference with a group of people in a resort setting – Hawaii, Mexico? Outdoorsy and tropical – big white frame buildings – rural.

We are outdoors near a field, and across the way I see an 18-wheeler pulling a flatbed containing a gigantic cage crammed with circus animals. They are starting to escape, and as I watch, the bars on the cage break, and the animals rush out.

We are all across the field and behind a barbed wire fence, but now I notice there is a hole in the fence. We start running for cover and (I think) manage to get inside in time.

Whew!! Escape from wild energy out of control. Just in time!!! You don't have to be Freud to wonder what primitive forces are about to take over. Over the years I had other dreams with similar energy, all ending with the forces subsiding prior to their getting loose in my world. I managed to get safely inside just in time!

It wasn't until I was in a situation where I met someone who seemed attractive and interesting to me that I felt the loss acutely. At that point, what had been just one of many other losses, having an emotional, sexual partner, took the foreground and screamed for attention. Fortunately, like Rose (Olivia Dukakis) in the movie *Moonstruck,** I was able to practice my own version – to myself, at least – of her great line, "I can't invite you in because I'm married and because I know who I am."

Rose's approach managed the immediate situation in a way that felt right to me, but it didn't solve the core issue. A brush with potential intimacy awakened feelings of loneliness and yearning that had been dormant through the trauma of life changes over the past few years. I was in touch with what I had been missing and could no longer ignore my feeling. When I tried to describe this jumble of feelings, here's what came to me:

> *Be reft*
> *I have just come across a new word: reft*
> *be*
> *reft*
> *if I were a composer I would write a piece*
> *or maybe*
> *if I were a writer*
> *I would elucidate it*
> *in short fiction or an essay*
> *or paint it*
> *seems like it would be easy*
> *but no*
> *all I can do*
> *is feel*
> *be*
> *reft*
> *with*
> *out*
> *hope*
> *companionship*
> *fun*
> *goofing around*
> *little asides*
> *making love*
> *being alone but not alone*
> *staying inside myself*
> *heft*
> *heft*
> *goes*
> *with*
> *reft*
> *as in heft the responsibility*
> *reft the responsibility*

take it
do it
keep on going
do what needs to be done
find the path
be here now
be reft.
                    Nina Krebs
                    April 2015

Bereft derives from bereave, roots of which are in Old English and German and have to do with deprivation, robbery, plundering, and even despoiling. To my surprise, I found reft is a real word. These feelings weighed me down. I couldn't recover and felt heavy and listless as I did my daily jobs.

Finally, with a little help from what I know about cognitive therapy*, and substantial self-confrontation, I moved forward. *Cognitive therapy*, pioneered by psychiatrist Albert Ellis, is based on a model, which states that thoughts, feelings and behavior are all connected. Individuals can move toward overcoming difficulties and meeting their goals by identifying and changing faulty thinking, problematic behavior, and distressing emotional responses. We have the capacity to create healthy responses to things that upset us rather than being controlled by old belief systems. I don't subscribe fully to this point of view, but it can be a helpful tool and was for me in this situation.

I assumed this sidetrack into fantasy romance was my unique experience. The people I knew who were in similar life situations seemed to go with the flow, manage their business along with that of their loved ones, and stay out of serious, life-disrupting trouble. One day I had lunch with friends who also cared for spouses with Alzheimer's. We were talking about loneliness and loss. We may even have been nudging toward issues of sleeping with our "loved ones" or not, and the resulting lack of intimacy. The word "sex" hadn't been spoken.

One woman said, "Yeah, when I say something to a man, and he adds to the conversation or asks a question, I hardly know what to say! My mouth just hangs open with surprise." We all nodded agreement.

We went on from there. One of the women said, "I was out for a walk on the trail the other day, and I saw a man coming toward me. As he approached and walked by me he said one word: 'Obsession.' That's the only perfume I've worn for years, and he recognized it. I was ready to drop my clothes right there!"

Though sexual deprivation takes its toll, it's the loss of intimacy and being known by another that digs the deepest chasm. What are the choices in a marriage to someone with dementia? Deprivation forever? An affair? Transcendence?

I sure don't know. My sense is that the person with dementia has no way to comprehend the loss of intimacy and reciprocity experienced by his or her spouse. And that doesn't begin to deal with their feelings of confusion and isolation. Even sleeping together with no prospect of sexual intimacy becomes problematic. People with Alzheimer's are not usually peaceful sleepers because they are restless and noisy.

Sleep deprivation had finally given me permission to make the move to my own bedroom. This was a huge relief, but this decision was yet another transition requiring careful, compassionate conversation. Part of that conversation was Dave's expression of loss. By this time he seemed comfortable with an affectionate relationship without benefits, but my move felt like one more injury to my partner's sense of self and wellbeing. For me, it was a loss of contact a last vestige of intimacy. My sleep improved, which helped me cope with daily life.

As an older woman, it's difficult for me to imagine an intimate relationship with a new partner. The thought of disrobing in the presence of another is enough to quell the idea. And yet, making a choice for eternal reft is more deprivation and plundering than I desire in my remaining time on the planet.

For her 50th wedding anniversary, my friend who had once been a travel agent and knew her way around the world, reserved a beautiful corner suite in an upscale hotel in downtown San Francisco. Her husband's Alzheimer's had been diagnosed, but he was conversant. They arrived in "The Golden City" on a glorious day, and Janeane was excited about being there and about celebrating her wonderful marriage.

They walked into the luxurious suite. She felt disappointed. She remembered earlier times Bill had sent flowers even though his memory was going, but she was happy to be in the beautiful surroundings. Bill said, "This is nice," slipped off his street clothes, put on his PJs and crawled into bed. He pulled the blankets up to his nose and was asleep almost instantly. Janeane fished her Kindle out of her tote and read for a while. She decided to go for a walk. There was plenty of time before they would go to dinner.

When she returned to the hotel she suggested Bill get up. He reluctantly agreed. Janeane showered and donned the dress she had thoughtfully selected for this special occasion. She loved the place they planned to dine, and expected Bill would perk up at dinnertime. This was a spot they had enjoyed together many times over the years. The maître d' seated them at a choice table in the corner of the dimly-lit dining room. The setting couldn't have been more romantic. Bill reached for the oversized menu as the waiter began to place it in front of him. He held it upside down and opened it. He looked at Janeane, frowning with confusion, "Where are we?" he asked.

"At our favorite restaurant in San Francisco!" she answered feeling surprised.

"Couldn't we just eat at home?" he said. "Why are we here?"

Nothing improved throughout the weekend. They left early Sunday to return to the East Bay. Because of Bill's ingrained social skills and ability to function in his familiar home environment, Janeane had badly underestimated his level of impairment. Her wishes for one last romantic celebration had blurred her judgment in planning the anniversary weekend.

Wedding anniversaries are especially poignant because they emphasize the loss of partnership and romance. Holidays in general are difficult. Each has its special history, mythology, memories, and connections. It is weird to be in the company of someone with whom you have shared decades of Thanksgivings with their successes and mishaps, and he can barely focus on today's dinner.

Many of us have old wounds about holidays that surface on those special days when we think we should enjoy ourselves. We need to stay mindful and separate the past from the present in order to appreciate good things happening around us. A partner with dementia brings up new scenarios of pain. In the days preceding a recent Thanksgiving, I had a hard time getting excited about the fun our family was planning. Things were going well, the weather was glorious, and I should have been having a good time but wasn't. I realized that this would probably be the last Thanksgiving Dave would recognize us.

Because of his heart condition, the possibility of each holiday being his last has haunted our family for several years. This year felt different. I could see Dave fading, being less aware and less able to follow conversations than this time the year before. In addition to whatever else they are, holidays are markers. On that Thanksgiving Thursday, I wanted it to be Friday. I walked to the park and went through my Qigong practice, breathing deeply, trying to release my heavy feelings. That helped a little, but I wondered how I would get through the day.

I deeply love my family. Karen and her husband had been working on dinner since Monday, I had invited a guest, and Spencer was excited about the big holiday leading up to his birthday a few days later. I'm not sure that Dave was tracking Thanksgiving at all, despite conversations about it and decorations at Meadow.

I had made no plans to bring Dave home with me after family dinner at Karen's as I had done the year before for Thanksgiving, Christmas, and New Year's. That current plan was good thinking on my part. I picked Dave up at Meadow around 1:30, and he was back there by 7:30. Dinner was the best ever. Although I felt very, very sad, I loved being with the family and was able to get through the day in a good enough way.

Seeing Dave lost and confused in a holiday setting mitigated the fun and fantasy associated with celebration. On one hand I would prefer to avoid the situation completely, but that would be a huge loss, too. My feelings of love, gratitude, and loyalty to the clan prevent me from running away. My inner conflict immobilized me, and I was grateful that all I had to do was be there. My responsibility for making things work was tiny. Blessings come in small packages.

Loss of the simple enjoyment and romance of partnership, especially one based on these two aspects as well as other strong elements, can't be measured. At times, the only redeeming facet is a sense of humor. Here's a story Melissa shared with me a few years ago as I was stepping into the Alzheimer's alcove:

Jane and her husband, Dale, were in their late seventies and he had been diagnosed several years earlier. Historically, Dale had always been a jealous husband, accusing Jane of carrying on with other men whenever she attended an out of town conference. Even after he was in assisted living, Jane and Dale were able to maintain an active sex life and proceeded to make love one night after going to bed. When it was over, Dale said, "I'd better call Jane and tell her I'm going to be late." Jane's ears pricked up and she responded by saying, "What's she going to think about you being here with me like this?" Dale replied, "Oh, I'm not going to tell her!!" Jane quietly said, "Dale, turn on the light." He did and looked at her and said, "Are you Jane?"

Yes, humor is a huge part of self-care because it may not erase pain, but it offers distance and a bit of perspective. I tend to fall short in this dimension, but things certainly go better when I can lighten up.

Accepting loss and scaling down wants and expectations is the hardest part of self-care for me, but that reality check nourishes my energy and capacity to enjoy life with its limits now. Indulgent as I may feel at times, focus on self-care rather than on what I miss from my old life, strengthens and enriches me.

CHAPTER 13

Nina's Artful Dwelling
2017

About the time I settled into something that felt like my life, pressure for the next tectonic shift pulsated and rumbled beneath me. In retrospect, I know that the decision to move Dave to assisted living was organic, emerging in its own time, but it didn't feel that way when it happened. A major life transition, striated with self-questioning and assorted anxieties had jammed together abruptly after months of uncertainty.

What did I want next in my life now that I was relieved of 24/7 caregiving?

Decision making, financial planning, providing emotional support, and the physical work involved in Dave's move had commandeered my attention and energy over the past months, squeezing out time, energy, and space needed to muse about my future. Almost superstitiously, I had focused on the tasks at hand, ignoring occasional hopes and concerns about my next moves.

The holidays were approaching, then Dave's birthday, as well as long-planned visits from people who live far away. No convenient time for my move, if there is such a thing, screamed at me from the calendar. When I moved, it would be my third full household move in four years, not counting transfers of significant bulk in and out of a studio and a storage unit.

Initially, my motivation centered on practical matters like finding a smaller, less expensive place within walking distance of things I needed. To-move or not-to-move questions hovered. I didn't feel a strong pull either way. Early in the year 2017, my interest and energy for moving increased. I began driving around likely neighborhoods and searching Craig's List and Zillow to acquaint myself with current rental market in the Walnut Creek/Pleasant Hill area. Karen was knowledgeable about neighborhoods and the housing market, and she jumped in to help me. I could imagine moving sometime before summer.

Rarely in my life had I been this befuddled about what I wanted. I knew I needed to give myself some time, and even though I had identified my hopes and wishes about the move, I wasn't making much headway.

In January 2017, I received an unexpected gift. I attended the same workshop, *Artist's Eye-Writer's Voice** I had participated in the previous year in Pt. Reyes. It was at that workshop the year before that I had decided to write this book about my caregiver experience. This time the little journey to the coast was much simpler than it had been the previous year because Dave was safely at Meadow, and I didn't have to arrange every minute of his care while I was away. I anticipated a relaxing weekend with focus on writing and visual art in the company of writers and artists.

The writing instructor mentioned that she was working on a new book about women writers at the end of their lives and the dwellings that they chose or designed for themselves. A window opened for me. My move could be a creative project, an art installation, in fact, not just a lockstep practical decision with no emotional juice. I could design a space that soothed and inspired me. Now I was motivated. I could hardly wait to get home to start house hunting.

The rental market in the Bay Area was tight, pricey, and fast moving, making it absolutely necessary for me to be clear about what I wanted and prepared to decide and act quickly when I found it. I made a list to help clarify my wants and needs and began to think about my move in concrete terms. I wasn't yet clear about whether it would be a single dwelling or in some kind of complex, but I knew my main criteria.

Karen and I researched many places, visited several, talked with property owners, and clarified the location I hoped for. Juggling location, price, dwelling type, aesthetics, availability, and parking challenged our tenacity and judgment. It's like choosing a life partner. How do you know it's going to work until you try it? Close to resignation, thinking I would have to spend the entire spring looking for a place to live, an invisible hand guided me home. I "accidentally" landed in the right place at the right time, checked out a condo I had formerly rejected, and with Karen's support, said, "I'll take it!"

March 1, 2017, I received the keys to my new dwelling in a huge complex in Walnut Creek, The Keys, which had been built in the '70's as a place for swinging singles, or that's how the story goes. Despite its reputation and the fact that a good number of the original residents were still in place, my chosen complex seemed neither swinging nor single-oriented. Residents were friendly, ethnically diverse, of varied ages and family constellations, all of which made me feel at home.

Three busy, company-filled weeks passed between the day I secured the condo and the move. Since I had downsized twice previously, I couldn't imagine packing would be too challenging, especially since the condo had lots of storage, and I didn't have to perform the cruel chore of discarding things I loved. Melissa urged me to hire movers to pack my household goods in addition to moving the big items, but since I thought I could pack everything in a week, I ignored her advice.

With Dave at Meadow, I had free rein to disband the duplex and stack boxes. I began with fine china, books, and art supplies that I wouldn't need for a while and worked forward into the realm of everyday objects. I had told the movers I would be moving twenty boxes. One hundred would have been a better guess. I'm deeply grateful to all those who came to help: Karen, Judy, Margaret, Rachel, Lynn, and in the crunch, Erica and Rex. Nearly every day before the move, someone was there helping me, not only with physical labor but with moral support in the face of my feeling overwhelmed.

When the day arrived for movers to fetch my stuff, I was close to ready and excited. I went outdoors to open the gate and welcome the movers. As I opened the front door, I glanced down and to my horror saw a dead mourning dove on the lawn, practically under my feet. The poor thing lying on its side with its little feet curled up appeared innocent and vulnerable. Dead. I took a breath. What did it mean? Was it a sign? It couldn't be on this day of excitement and new beginning. I'm not superstitious; I am a scientist. It was a dead bird. True, and, yet, as it happens, I had spent years researching shamanism, native connections with nature, and the prominence of birds as spiritual symbols. I couldn't unsee the little corpse.

I was already dealing with the strangeness of moving into a place of my choice that I could set up exactly the way I wanted, at what felt like Dave's expense. Uncanny feelings of apprehension and guilt crept in. It had been hard for me to sustain good feelings and excitement about the move, although I had been working toward this goal for a long time. Just as it was coming together, the dead bird's image of spiritual disconnection felt like a kick in the stomach.

I went inside and picked up the fireplace shovel and some paper towels. I gently placed the bird in the organic trash container, trying not to shudder. Providing such an unceremonious resting place for the remains mirrored my mixed, morbid feelings. When I went inside, I didn't say anything about the bird to Rachel who was wrapping and packing at warp speed, but I couldn't erase the image of the perfect dead dove. As much as I didn't want to harbor it, a sense of impending darkness hovered. I dismissed feelings of doom as remnants of exhaustion and stress.

The movers were on time and knew what they were about. After the big moving truck was situated and the ramp in place, three guys set to work shrink wrapping and blanketing my worldly possessions and moving them onto the truck. They must have all been physics majors because they knew about angles and balance points and maneuvered big chunks of furniture with seeming ease until all the rooms were empty.

Rachel had spent the last two days and nights with me, organizing and packing as we talked and listened to music. Her company and support made progress possible, much faster and less tedious than if I had been slogging through it on my own. She had also helped at the condo, moving and assembling shelves in the walk-in closet, and doing as much work as we could in the storage unit. She left around noon on moving day when she could see that the movers were nearing completion.

By mid-afternoon the furniture and boxes were all at the condo, not in the orderly way I had imagined because the storage unit, which was to hold rarely used items wasn't yet available. My color-coordinated signs and box labels had worked to an extent, but not as well as I had planned. In the vacated duplex dirt had accumulated over the past three years in unexposed areas under beds and behind dressers; all those dust bunnies and missing hair clips came out. The saving grace was that I had nearly two weeks to sort, finish packing, and clean. I reminded myself that I had planned it that way, could easily empty and clean one room per day and still have time remaining before my lease was up.

The big move had been accomplished! At least my possessions had changed addresses, but now I faced mountain ranges of boxes, bags, and misshapen bundles in every available space at the condo. I still confronted unpacking as well as shopping for the household items I would need to finish the move. I planned to wind up the physical move before I began changing mailing addresses and cancelling services at the old address.

My friend Lynn arrived late in the afternoon of moving day, and although I was stressed and exhausted, we began organizing. The next day, Saturday, she took over setting up the kitchen and was able to complete that job, a practical port in a sea of chaos. I organized my bedroom and had one comfortable, habitable space. The guest room/studio was stacked with boxes from floor to ceiling. Lynn graciously agreed to sleep on the sofa in the living room, which also huddled amidst a barricade of containers.

Lynn and I were congratulating ourselves when the phone rang, and I saw Jim Leehan's name on the caller ID. I assumed it was Melissa, and said, "Hi, Girlfriend," when I answered.

"No, it's me," Jim said. He sounded horrible. "I have terrible news," he said.

Melissa had collapsed and died.

Jim described the sequence of the day: Melissa's recognition that she might be having a heart attack. They went through two separate rounds with EMTs who read normal EKGs. They had been out shopping and when given the choice, they decided to go home, partly because it was closer, instead of to the hospital. Later that day, as Jim was driving Melissa, at her request, to have her nails done, a very Melissa-like thing to do when she wasn't feeling well, she had a final heart attack. She died before she was in the ambulance on the way to the hospital.

Lynn was with me when I received the news, and as I broke down, she held and comforted me, a true friend, still in grief from her husband's death less than a year earlier. I cried like I hadn't cried in years - can't even remember when. I couldn't imagine my world without Melissa, my friend and confidante for nearly 50 years. She had been with me through all the hard spots of my journey, and over recent months we had talked at least twice a week as I struggled through the decision about Dave's move to Meadow. At the same time, she and Jim were facing the challenge of leaving their beautiful home in Santa Fe to move to California for Jim's health.

Melissa had been excited that we would finally live in the same state, and yet, she was overwhelmed with the logistics and complexities of planning and executing a move. In one of our conversations, when it was clear that she was delaying her own care and taking on too much, I had urged Melissa to deal with her health concerns. "I don't want you to die before we get to live in the same state!" I told her, half-joking.

And then she died.

Images of the dead bird floated into my awareness from time to time. Even though I had tried to ignore it, the power of its placement was undeniable to me. It had put me on alert. I was not completely surprised by Jim's call, and that little bit of reserve generated by a warning sign, superstitious or not, sustained me as I moved numbly through the next few days.

The move wasn't nearly as finished as I had hoped. Far more debris remained in the old house than I had anticipated, dregs of living in every room. Items I had planned to dispose of were everywhere. I could barely think or move at this point, but I didn't want to leave the place in its current state. The landlords who had always been fair and supportive were anxious to get in to clean and paint. I knew I had to deal with the remains.

After I learned that Melissa's funeral would be the following Friday, I pulled my plans together. I sent out an SOS. Family and friends assembled and spent a day finishing my move out of the duplex. I wasn't much help. By late afternoon, everything had been moved into the condo and the space was clean enough to leave. I left instructions for the landlords to haul the remaining junk and charge me accordingly, which they did in a very fair way.

I told Dave what had happened. He responded with shock and sadness. Later, when I told him I was going to Santa Fe, he said, "Tell Jim and Missy hello for me, and that I'm sorry I can't be there too." I told him about Melissa's death again. And again. Then I decided if the subject came around another time, I would just let it go.

The funeral was Friday at St. Bede's Episcopal Church in Santa Fe. It was perfect. Melissa would have loved it. The only disconnect was that I couldn't call her and talk about it afterward.

I have few journal entries for the next few weeks. In my grief-laden state, I began doing what I could to unpack and organize my new home, not expecting much from myself. Time blurred. Judy was in and out, present and helpful. Karen showed up with support in the form of time for pedicures and lunch, unobtrusively checking in. Other family and friends were in touch. I took daily walks and went through the motions of Qigong. I managed my responsibilities with Dave and took care of the banking, bills, and other daily tasks.

Through my fog I hoped to have the condo in order by the time I flew off to the Long Island Guitar Festival, April 4. I almost made it. Time in New York at the festival, being roommates at the hotel where I have stayed many times with my other best friend, Karen Davis, fabulous music and the fun of the festival did its good work. I relaxed and absorbed the sweet respite from grief, moving and Dave-care.

The flight home dragged. I paid homage to the pioneers when my butt and knees screamed with seatitis and then, I got up, walked and stretched. My midnight drive home from Oakland International Airport was easy. I unlocked the door to my new home and slipped inside. Echoes of loss for Dave and Melissa resonated through me. Over that dark stream, despite my grief, I sensed a sprinkle of excitement about the new life I was unveiling.

I regained a guarded sense of habitual optimism. I was not bouncy, but I was better. Even when I couldn't accomplish much, I had established the routine of walking in the morning at least two miles and practicing Qigong in the park. In the early summer I had found a vibraphone teacher and began taking time almost every day for a full hour's practice on my vibraphone. This time-consuming routine felt fulfilling and satisfying to the point of being indulgent because it took nearly three hours every day. I worked at convincing myself I was worth it and needed these activities to recover from grief and to manage my stress level. Sticking to this plan required discipline. I was proud of myself for being able to maintain the routine and feel the benefit of the work.

I compared my life with the previous summer, and the difference in my sense of wellbeing contrasted from grainy black and white to Technicolor. Fantasies of driving my car off a cliff had evaporated as had the wish that I could get on the freeway and just keep driving. When I opened my eyes in the morning, I usually felt happy and looked forward to the day. I loved my new living space, the aesthetics of the condo complex, and its proximity to downtown. It felt right to me, attractive and comfortable.

I had begun to enjoy life much as I had before *The Clamp* gripped me. I attended events or went out to eat without Dave. Now I found myself feeling happier and appreciating more than ever the things I love doing. I didn't take them for granted. I treasured ordinary moments, including spending time with family. I enjoyed phone conversations or visits with friends as special occasions, not just commonplace events. I practiced attending to what I was doing and engaging it fully rather than thinking about all the other things I might or ought to be doing. I was able to accomplish the routine work that is part of ordinary life and take care of Dave in the ways that were still necessary. The grasp of *The Clamp* had begun to ease, but it had not disappeared.

I felt the constraint of *The Clamp* most when making plans with friends. Everyone has scheduling guidelines, but since mine were mainly about Dave's schedule, not mine, I would occasionally forget and then need to rearrange. Or my windows to plan events made it difficult to match times with the availability of others. A sense of impending responsibility, being on call, hovered near me much of the time. This heightened when Dave started calling me at random times, like at midnight, 5:30 A. M. or 5 minutes after I had just talked with him or returned home from a visit to Meadow. By this time *The Clamp* was a heavy wrap on a summer day. I would mindfully leave it at home only to find myself clamped again.

My growing friendship with Joanie as we had supported each other's decision to place our husbands in assisted living was a gift. It helped to check in with another person who was facing similar challenges. We talked about our mixed feelings of grief, guilt, and relief. We visited our husbands together at Meadow, which eased the caregiver pressures and anticipatory grief we both experienced. We coordinated lunch dates with the men and shared driving tasks for LARC.

Late one afternoon, I was walking after I had a good day. I found myself feeling cautious about how good I felt. A vague feeling that something was about to happen agitated me. I confronted myself for this catastrophic thinking and let the thought go. I reflected on how traumatizing caregiving had been and continued to be in a less concentrated way. It would take time and intention to work it through.

My friend Lynn and I had been talking over the past three years about going to the beach or the mountains for a getaway, but we had never found a good time for the trip. Finally in June 2017 we had made plans to meet in Point Reyes, a picturesque, rugged ocean-side art community perched on the coast of Marin County. I packed my car with carefully selected food, hiking gear, art supplies, writing material, and even my music lesson in case I had time to review it.

I arrived at the Bovine Bakery in Point Reyes exactly on time at 11:00 in the morning. Lynn was not there yet. I texted her and she replied that she would be at the bakery in five minutes. I went across the street and around the block to the public restroom. On exiting the bathroom I tripped over a divider curb in the parking lot and landed hard on my left wrist.

When I looked at my wrist, I knew it was broken. It looked like a blue python that had swallowed a rat. My arm was swollen, discolored, and misshapen. I supported my broken wrist with my right hand, struggled to my feet and started slowly to return to the Bovine Bakery. I was woozy but quite sure I could make it across the street and reseat myself on the bench at the bakery. I saw that Lynn had not yet arrived. Two women resting on a nearby bench asked if I were okay. "No," I said. "I think I have broken my wrist." They offered to get me water. Shortly, the cashier from the bakery appeared with a bag of ice. Within minutes Lynn arrived.

Lynn efficiently and calmly went for my car. She grabbed my clothes bag, cosmetic kit, and pillow. We got directions to the local clinic and headed there in her car. We learned that we would need to proceed to Marin General Hospital in San Rafael, which the GPS told us was 46 minutes away. Three hours after we arrived at the hospital I was released, my arm in a splint, and a prescription for pain meds in my good hand. I convinced Lynn to go on her way with her friends. Shortly after she left, Karen and Spencer picked me up outside the emergency room and drove me home to Walnut Creek in rush hour traffic.

I have never been as thrilled to see home. My arm throbbed and I hurt all over. Karen said I was still ghostly white. I could hardly wait to stretch out on my bed. Nine-year-old Spencer had overheard his mother say that I needed to have a snack along with my pain pills. He said, "Grandma, I'll fix you a snack before you take your pills." He proceeded to peel me an orange, which he served along with a cookie and mango juice. He stood beside my chair and said, "I suggest you drink all your juice and swallow your pill." His sincerity and concern touched me and raised my spirits.

It took an extraordinary amount of energy to accomplish the simple task of informing Dave about my injury, and I was glad that I was able to do it. A couple of days after the fall Judy went with me to have dinner with him at Meadow. Her presence and support helped. Once again I was grateful that I had made the decision to place Dave in assisted living rather than trying to care for him at home.

I needed to arrive at Kaiser for my surgery appointment at 8:10 A.M. Friday, June 30, 2017. Karen took me to the hospital where Erica waited for us. Admission for surgery went smoothly including my conversation with the surgeon who assured me I would regain full use of my hand. I had been very worried about that as well as other aspects of surgery at age 78. Surgery went well, and I spent the next few days resting and recovering.

This broken-wing experience brought me face-to-face with the fragility of my own aging process, which has been concurrent with Dave's decline into Alzheimer's. I had fallen hard twice in the past month. I can no longer count on my capacity to handle all that comes my way or depend on my ability to bounce back quickly. I decided these breaks, both my wrist and the time off, were metaphors for this chapter in my life. Any of us can trip and face an unexpected set of circumstances, problems to be solved, and possibly, opportunities. How we recover is key.

I felt grateful for my loved ones who were affectionate, attentive, and helpful throughout the entire ordeal. Lynn and I revisited Pt. Reyes a year later. The irony of my situation didn't evade me. I lived where I had yearned to be for years and had my very own place that I loved in the Bay Area. The purple cast on my arm reminded me that life is fragile and impermanent. I trusted my wrist would recover, and I would go about life with fresh awareness and humility.

I renewed my commitment to doing the things that were important to me.

CHAPTER 14

Good Night, Dave
I Love You

Journal entry: Saturday, January 21, 2017 – the day of the Women's March

Dave just called from Meadow as he does about this time every night "Just to hear your voice," he says. I told him about going to Berkeley to the annual luncheon with my Qigong class and about walking around the UC Berkeley campus with a friend from the group. We had our usual conversation about events at Meadow and what he could remember from his day. I'm happy to hear energy in his voice and to picture him at a younger, healthier time.

He's telling me about activities he attended during the day, and then something a little different slips into the conversation. He said, "And a bunch of us were sitting around at dinner talking about our lives before, and what we did for work. It's a way of getting to know each other. We just sat there shooting the bull until the staff kicked us out."

He hesitates here and there, waiting for a word, but in a limited way, he sounds like the old Dave whose extraordinary skills ushered people into conversations they didn't know they could have. Remnants of those skills remain, perhaps, and he and his compatriots at Meadow are opening doors of connection.

He added that "the group" was talking about things they appreciated at Meadow: the staff, the food, and that it was a good place to be.

I asked if any of the staff people were in on the conversation, and he said, "Not until they came to kick us out of the dining room."

"Next time," he said, "we could talk about things we would like to see happen here and make suggestions for things we would like to do."

I said, "It sounds like you are using your well-honed skills to help
people get to know and support each other."
"And I think they appreciate it," he said.

This snippet reminded me of what used to be and felt both heartwarming and excruciating. Chances were good that by the next day, or even the next minute, he would have no recollection of that conversation. The good news was that it happened, he remembered it long enough to tell me, and it indicated Dave and others in this environment away from a traditional home were opening possibilities for community and mutual support.

Finishing our phone call, I complimented and encouraged Dave, and he moved into his mantra about how much he loved me, how lucky he was to have me in his life, how the girls I and were the greatest gifts he ever had, and how he didn't want to be a burden on me.

I felt my heart seize, and I centered myself to accept his offering, respond, and move toward the end of our conversation. What should feel like love, felt like a rose-covered *Clamp*. I wanted to find a way to hear and support him and let the energy flow through me rather than feeling like I had received a blow to my solar plexus. Guilt, pain, and a feeling of being pummeled by repetition let me know I couldn't give him what he wanted and survive. I directed the conversation onto a partnership path and pointed out that coincidentally he spent time with his group, and I spent time with mine. Even though we were in different places, we were continuing our lives in the way we always had.

Then we could say, "Goodnight. I love you!"

When I tell people about these conversations, they say, "You are lucky!"

In a way that is absolutely true. It doesn't feel good though, to be the center of Dave's life, which seems to be his view of me. He doesn't make demands on me directly or guilt trip me verbally, but there is a way I feel like I fail him because I can't be there for him in the way he wishes.

Dave has always been expressive about his love for me, which many women long for, and I appreciated. Now, though, the words feel rote and heavy, like a chain he wraps around me and pulls tight. I can thank him and tell him I love him, but hard as I try to summon the feeling, my words are empty. I am sad that he relies on me for his sense of self because I can't possibly be that for him. I can't save him.

We all face our endings in different ways. In his book, *Being Mortal: Illness, Medicine and What Matters in the End,** Atul Gawande addresses end-of-life issues. We need to learn about this process while we can make conscious choices rather than thinking magic will happen, and we will live in healthy body and mind forever.

My life improved significantly within a week of Dave's move because I was less vigilant, sleeping better, able to meditate and exercise, and I felt like I could relax and move around at home and in the world. People started telling me that I looked less stressed and 10 years younger. I felt lighter and didn't wake each day with a feeling of dread.

I had underestimated the positive impact living at Meadow would have on Dave. I had been engaged in my own survival and guilt, and the fact that he would actually be better off in an environment designed to care for him had escaped me. As time went on, I attempted to arrange his return from outings with me at a time that an activity that he enjoyed was in progress there. When he returned to Meadow, whoever was at the desk said, "Welcome back, Dave. We missed you!" and he shifted into being at home there. After seeing that happen a few times, I felt assured that his life was good in his new home, and even though he longed for me to be at his side, he was engaged with life in his space.

I confronted my challenges with aging and began recovering from the past few years' caregiving. I missed opportunities to do things I would enjoy because I assumed I wouldn't be able to follow through or it would be too much trouble to arrange. And then, sometimes too late, I remembered that was no longer the case. I COULD have gone to that opening or that concert. Even though I felt significant relief, Post Traumatic Stress continued just outside my awareness.

Becoming an unintended caregiver had changed my worldview. It didn't feel like it was something I could get over, even if I outlived Dave and had healthy years ahead of me. I can't predict or describe a personal outcome. Certainly I have acquired added layers of caution and vulnerability. Gratitude for my everyday life, humility and compassion for myself and others all feel strong as well.

I experienced early retirement syndrome all over again: I yearned to do more things simultaneously than would be possible for anyone. Then I would have to pause and sort them out. I was excited about my new-found freedom. I wanted to write, go out with friends, do Qigong, paint, hang out with Spencer, go to San Francisco, and play my vibraphone all at once. And I could imagine a trip to Mexico or New York in the process.

After a few months at Meadow, Dave's memory diminished and his gait seemed more halting. At times he was noticeably more confused than usual. His capacity for tracking, making sense of a schedule, or remembering what was going to happen next fell close to non-existent. Did these changes result from the move or were they predictable progress of Alzheimer's? Or both?

Dave was in a safe and nourishing place and was making peace with his life there. As he continued to decline, he had an option to move to memory care just down the hall. When my so-called friend had accused me of being seduced by the glamorous new facility at Meadow and said that I was only thinking of myself, not Dave, she had a point. I was thinking of Dave. He liked nice things and had always been particular about keeping his space clean and well-organized. But I also knew that if I walked into a depressing place every time I visited him, it would make it even harder for me to do what I needed to do.

My feelings about where he lived were important. If he were in some of the places Karen and I had checked out, every visit would have been an ordeal for me. As it was, when I walked into Meadow with its pretty, well-lighted reception area that opened onto a spacious living room and a view to the courtyard, I felt good. The environment did not add another layer of depression to this already difficult time. I could visit Dave there and be present, not spaced out just trying to maintain.

Despite confusion and disorientation, I could see that Dave's general mood and activity level were much improved. When I arrived unexpectedly at Meadow, he might be in his room watching sports on TV, but he was just as likely to be in the Activity Room participating in a game, discussion, or project with his peers. The trend of his adjustment was in the right direction, and my relief was proportional to that. Naturally, we both had ups and downs. I chose the ups!

Contrary to my hopes, I found that even though I was theoretically free to take short trips, I felt tethered. On one overnight in Sacramento visiting Judy, I received a call from Meadow and, based on the advice of the med tech there, decided to dash the 80 miles back to Walnut Creek and take Dave to the Emergency Room. He could have been taken by ambulance, or Karen could have helped out. I was concerned that if big decisions needed to be made, I should be the person doing that, not another family member. The least invasive or dramatic intervention for Dave was for me to step in. It turned out that Dave was released after extensive evaluation, and I returned him to Meadow just past midnight, six hours after his arrival at the emergency room.

Because of events like this, it's hard to make travel plans or even opt for a few days away. Nonetheless, I have taken several weeklong trips and a few shorter ones since Dave has been at Meadow, and when I am away I don't obsess about him. I have a hard time deciding to go in the first place because it feels simpler to stay put and be available if I am needed. I have vastly more freedom than I did before Dave moved, and I deeply appreciate it, but I still struggle to clarify how much responsibility is mine.

This story could have various endings. The question has remained, "How could both Dave and I make the most of our remaining time?"

I hadn't dared to think much about how I wanted my life to be for the next few years because taking care of Dave and managing our life together had been all-consuming. As opportunities emerged, I couldn't be sure what I would choose when I had the chance, but I felt highly motivated to enjoy whatever time I had left.

- I moved to a less expensive residence within walking distance of shops and only 10 minutes from Meadow via freeway.
- I spent time with family and friends, minus *The Clamp*, and in their environments rather than their having to visit me.
- For a long time I had wanted to travel with the seasons in a little RV taking time to write and paint along the way. Could I make this happen in some form? It would be hard to be away from my family for stretches of time, but I might find modified ways to pursue this fantasy.
- I began to take advantage of art, music and theater riches of the Bay Area, especially the San Francisco Symphony and the treasure-laden museums nearby.
- I had the option to check out classes available through a multitude of extension programs in different areas of interest.
- I began to greet each day as if I were a newborn babe and regard it with awe and gratitude. I could anticipate how I wanted to spend my time and usually carry through with my plans.

When I broke my wrist and had a bitter taste of vulnerability and mortality, I resolved even more solidly, not only to be mindful of where I was in time and space, but also to be thoughtful about my choices. We don't choose parts of what life brings us, but with hard work, we can decide how to live with our challenges.

I began to enjoy my reclaimed mobility and relinquish confining anxiety and tension. The following dream offered affirmation and a glimmer of direction:

Journal entry: December 12, 2016

I'm at an outdoor mall or park where there is an event going on – a big grassy square in front of Macy's and other stores. Friends (men) are seated at a table where they are handing out information or products for an organization or company. I stand off to the side, visiting with them when they are not busy.

Spencer is nearby and is watching and half-listening. Karen and Erica are around as well. There are lots of people enjoying the event, moving from place to place.

I am going on and on to everyone or to no one in particular about the level of commitment needed to learn a language or to play an instrument. And I am thinking, why would anyone do that? I am asking, "But what are the pleasures? What are the pleasures?" And I think about the joy of accomplishment, the pleasure of making music, the excitement of being able to converse in another language.

Before any discussion can happen, I see an extra-large, ivory-colored Hummer-like vehicle pull up in front of Macy's. Most of this monstrous machine is hidden behind a huge white tent, but under the edge of the tent, I see that it has let down a "foot" to steady it in place. On the foot nearest me, I see the Jaguar logo, and also Mac (as in Apple technology). Strange, I think, it looked like a Hummer when I saw it pass.

Attendants, lightly-bearded young men, all dressed in wheat-colored, tasseled tunics with slim pants, line up on two sides of the door and when it opens, a wizard in golden robes and a tall hat steps out, aided by the attendant closest to the door. He walks ceremoniously between the lined-up attendants, and then they spread out in a square in front of him, clearing a path as he ambles around the park.

I try to get out of the way, but every place I go the entourage is there first. I want to take photos, and I can't get an angle. I think the cadre is headed for the far corner of the park where a throne is centered on a dais.

Finally, I am outside of the entourage, looking at them as they approach. I am amazed to see that one of the attendants on my side of the group is a very tall Caucasian woman with a patch over one eye, dressed in the uniform of an Iranian soldier. She is quietly singing an American popular song in English as she walks along with the group. I am about to get an angle for my photo.

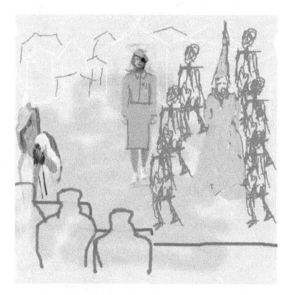

In the dream I had a hard time securing a good place to see and comprehend the wizard and his entourage. Who were they? Where did they come from in their big, expensive vehicle? Why did they show up now? What did they mean to me? I moved around until I ultimately found a place with a good angle for viewing the scene and taking photos.

I accepted my dream as a cosmic gift, affirmation of my tenacity, search for meaning, and willingness to move around in the world despite trouble finding my way. Magic is present in my life, visible and practically running over me. The wounded woman warrior is still marching and singing her own song. I will explore what I can learn from her and from the wizard. I hope you will do the same with insights that come to you.

Even as you support and tend the needs of your loved one, I invite you and encourage you to honor your inner guides. Seek and acknowledge your gifts for enjoying life.

To thine own self be true.

Patient.

And, compassionate.

Epilogue

Dave has been in assisted living for two and a half years. His spirits are good and he says he understands, that with his aging process, it is a good place for him to be. He knows our little family and me, but he gets mixed up about where we all live and who belongs with whom. His physical health, while fragile, far exceeds his doctors' predictions for him, which I attribute to his healthy living habits and the good care he receives at Meadow.

I find it painful to visit and spend time with Dave in his diminished capacity, especially when it is time to say goodbye and he is confused about where I live. "Don't you live here?" he asks as I walk toward the front door at Meadow. I am touched by his infinite love and support for me, and it hurts to see him compromised and vacant. I do the best I can to be a loving partner in a bad situation.

I am deeply grateful for family, friends and for the good life I have in my artful dwelling and the world at large.

Nina Krebs
August 2019

References

Alzheimer's Association. Legal issues related to elder care, (https://www.alz.org/help-support/caregiving/financial-legal-planning/planning-ahead-for-legal-matters)

Aortic stenosis. Aortic valve stenosis is a narrowing of the aortic valve in the heart, which reduces the amount of blood that can flow into the aorta. The aorta is the largest artery in the body. The aorta begins at the top of the left ventricle, the heart's muscular pumping chamber. The heart pumps blood from the left ventricle into the aorta through the aortic valve. When the valve narrows, the heart has to pump harder to push the same amount of blood, which may eventually weaken the heart.

The Artist's Eye, The Writer's Voice. Mesa Refuge, Point Reyes Station, CA. A weekend workshop I attended January 2015 and 2016 that profoundly influenced my decision to write this book. Facilitated by Elizabeth Fischel and Susan Tillett.

Attorney-locater. https://www.alz.org/help-support/caregiving/financial-legal-planning/planning-ahead-for-legal-matters. Contact your local Alzheimer's Association chapter or use our online Community Resource Finder. Use the online directory of the National Academy of Elder Law Attorneys. Visit the Eldercare Locator online or call 800.677.1116. Visit LawHelp.org to learn about free or reduced cost legal aid programs in your community.

Be Here Now. Published by Lama Foundation, 1978. Ram Dass (born Richard Alpert; April 6, 1931) an American spiritual teacher put forth his philosophy in this book. He is known for his personal and professional associations with Timothy Leary at Harvard University in the early 1960s, for his travels to India and his relationship with the Hindu guru Neem Karoli Baba. Ram Dass now resides on Maui, where he shares his teachings through the Internet and through bi-yearly retreats on Maui. His work continues to be a path of inspiration to his old students and friends as well as young people who are just discovering the path of *Be Here Now.*

Codependent. The codependent (enabler) person feels worthless unless they are needed by, and making sacrifices for, the patient or needy one. The enabler gets satisfaction from anticipating and meeting the partner's needs and is only happy when making sacrifices for their partner. They feel they must be needed by this other person to be worthwhile or have a purpose in life. See Nepo. Mark. *The Book of Awakening: Having the Life You Want by Being Present to the Life You Have,* Conari Press, May 2000, entry for March 18.

Cognitive therapy is based on a model, which states that thoughts, feelings, and behavior are all connected, and that individuals can move toward overcoming difficulties and meeting their goals by identifying and changing unhelpful or inaccurate thinking, problematic behavior, and distressing emotional responses. This involves the individual working collaboratively with the therapist to develop skills for testing and modifying beliefs, identifying distorted thinking, relating to others in different ways, and changing behaviors. Psychiatrist Albert Ellis pioneered this approach.

Compartmentalization is a psychological defense mechanism that helps us keep conflicting feelings or ideas separated in our consciousness, a form of emotional tunnel vision. For example: A person who is very religious and also a scientist holds the opposing beliefs in different cognitive compartments, such that when they are in church, they can have blind faith, but when they are in the laboratory, they question everything.

Downwinder syndrome refers to cancer that affected individuals and communities in the intermountain area between the Cascade and Rocky Mountain ranges primarily in Arizona, Nevada, and Utah but also in Oregon, Washington, and Idaho who were exposed to radioactive contamination or nuclear fallout from atmospheric or underground nuclear weapons testing, and nuclear accidents.

FINE. Fucked up, Insecure, Neurotic and Egotistical is author Louise Penny's definition in her novel *Fatal Grace* "I'm FINE…" Penny, Louise. *Fatal Grace,* St. Martin's Press, 2011.

Friedan, Betty. *The Feminine Mystique,* New York, W. W. Norton & Company, 1963.

Gawande, Atul. *Being Mortal: Illness, Medicine and What Matters in the End,* Metropolitan Books/Henry Holt & Company, 2014.

Grounding. A term used to describe a process of relaxing in order to focus and tune into one's emotional state. Grounding is an important element in maintaining a balanced and connected mind-body-spirit existence.

Inner guide or inner self. The inner self is an individual's personal internal identity, one that is distinct from identities defined by external, social forces and relationships. It is closely linked to a person's values, beliefs, goals and motivations. The term also implies a level of authenticity not associated with external identities and labels; it is the "true self."

Iris. A movie starring Judy Dench and Kate Winslet, directed by Richard Eyre, written by Charles Wood, Richard Eyre, Miramax Films, 2001. There is also a later version.

Kaiser Permanente. Kaiser Permanente is a health care system that evolved from industrial health care programs for construction, shipyard, and steel mill workers for the Kaiser industrial companies during the late 1930s and 1940s. It was opened to public enrollment in July 1945 and continues to be a major healthcare provider.

Krebs, Nina Boyd. Books include: *Changing Woman Changing Work,* Macmurray and Beck Communication, 1993; with Robert Allen *Dramatic Psychological Story Telling: Using Psychotheatrics and the Expressive Arts,* Palgrave Macmillan, 2006; *Edgewalkers: Defusing Cultural Boundaries on the New Global Frontier,* New Horizon Press, 1999; with Robert Allen, *Psychotheatrics, the New Art of Self-Transformation,* Garland Press, (now Scholarly Title) 1979.

Levaquin (levofloxacin) is a fluoroquinolone antibiotic that fights bacteria in the body.

Mild to moderate generalized atrophy with minimal scattered presumed microangiopathic ischemic changes in the cerebral white matter. This is the language used to describe the changes in Dave's brain structure that indicated he was suffering from "Alzheimer's-like symptoms." It means that the MRI revealed observable changes to the brain that could explain changes in Dave's memory and behavior.

Moonstruck. A 1987 movie about a family in Brooklyn, starring Cher, Nicholas Cage, Danny Aiello, and Olivia Dukakis. Directed by Norman Jewison.

Narcissism. I am referring more to "narcissistic style" than to narcissistic personality disorder (NPD). However, this definition from Wikipedia is helpful. People with NPD are characterized by their persistent grandiosity, excessive need for admiration, and a personal disdain and lack of empathy for other people. As such, the person with NPD usually displays arrogance and a distorted sense of superiority, and they seek to establish abusive power and control over others. Self-confidence (a strong sense of self) is different from narcissistic personality disorder. A person with narcissistic personality disorder usually exhibits a fragile ego (self concept), intolerance of criticism, and a tendency to belittle others in order to validate their own superiority.

Narcissistic defenses. Inability to accept feedback that clashes with one's sense of self. Inability to acknowledge feelings of emptiness or personal neediness. High levels of personal achievement and patina of being special may cover feelings of insecurity or neediness.

O'Rourke, Meghan. *The Long Goodbye, a memoir,* New York, Riverhead Books, the Penguin Group, 2011, page 131.

Palliative care. Palliative care is a multidisciplinary approach to specialized medical and nursing care for people with life-limiting illnesses. It focuses on providing relief from the symptoms, pain, physical stress and mental stress of a terminal diagnosis. The goal is to improve quality of life for both the person and their family.

Physician Orders for Life-Sustaining Treatment (POLST) is a document that gives seriously-ill patients more control over their end-of-life care, including medical treatment, extraordinary measures (such as a ventilator or feeding tube) and CPR. Printed on bright pink paper, and signed by both a patient and physician, nurse practitioner or physician assistant, POLST can prevent unwanted or ineffective treatments, reduce patient and family suffering, and ensure that a patient's wishes are honored.

Payable on Death (POD). A POD or payable on death account is a type of account that is an arrangement between a bank or credit unit and an account holder that designates beneficiaries to receive a person's account upon the death of the account holder. To create a POD account, the account holder will have to fill out the proper paperwork at the bank or credit union where they have an account.

Power of attorney. (POA) A power of attorney is a legal document that allows someone to make decisions for you, or act on your behalf, if you're no longer able to make decisions or if you no longer want to make your own decisions.

Plaques and tangles in the brain. Dementia researchers are focused on the role of two proteins: *Plaques.* Beta-amyloid is a leftover fragment of a larger protein. When these fragments cluster together, they appear to have a toxic effect on neurons and to disrupt cell-to-cell communication. These clusters form larger deposits called amyloid plaques, which also include other cellular debris. *Tangles.* Tau proteins play a part in a neuron's internal support and transport system to carry nutrients and other essential materials. In Alzheimer's disease, tau proteins change shape and organize themselves into structures called neurofibrillary tangles. The tangles disrupt the transport system and are toxic to cells. https://www.mayoclinic.org/diseases-conditions/alzheimers-disease/symptoms-causes/syc-20350447

Russo, Francine. *"The Givers,"* *Scientific American Mind,* November/December 2016, pp.28-35.) *"The Caregiver's Dilemma," Scientific American Mind,* November/December 2016, page 28.

Saijo, Albert. Saijo was a poet of the Beat Generation. Reference to the poem in the text can be found on the Internet at https://peopleplanningandpoetry.wordpress.com/2016/06/22/bodhisattva-vows-by-albert-saijo/

Self-reflecting other. A term from intersubjective theory in psychology used to describe the interaction of one person with another. The subject person sees herself or himself reflected in the object person, thus creating a sense of being known and understood. Among the early authors who explored Intersubjective systems theory in psychoanalysis, in an explicit or implicit way, were Heinz Kohut, Robert Stolorow, George E. Atwood, Jessica Benjamin in the United States, and Silvia Montefoschi in Italy.

Transcatheter Aortic Valve Replacement (TAVR). For high risk aortic stenosis patients, TAVR surgery may be an option that provides an aortic valve repair without the physical stress of open-heart surgery. The procedure is performed by inserting instruments into the femoral artery through a small incision and gently advancing through the blood vessels until the aortic valve is reached. For the TAVR procedure, the artificial valve is bundled into a tiny package that is small enough to be moved through the blood vessel along with the instruments. When in place, the valve replacement is deployed, opening to its full size. Once the TAVR is in place, it controls the release of blood from the heart. (www.verywell.com)

Tropinin level. A troponin test measures the levels troponin T or troponin I proteins in the blood. These proteins are released when the heart muscle has been damaged, such as occurs with a heart attack. The more damage there is to the heart, the greater the amount of troponin T and I there will be in the blood.

Whittaker, Carl. Co-author with Augustus Napier. *The Family Crucible: The Intense Experience of Family Therapy,* Harper Perennial, 1988.

Notes from the Alzheimer's Association
(https://www.alz.org)

- Dementia is not a specific disease. It's an overall term that describes a group of symptoms associated with a decline in memory or other thinking skills severe enough to reduce a person's ability to perform everyday activities. Alzheimer's disease accounts for 60 to 80 percent of cases.
- An estimated 5.7 million Americans of all ages are living with Alzheimer's dementia in 2018. This number includes an estimated 5.5 million people age 65 and older and approximately 200,000 individuals under age 65 who have early-onset Alzheimer's.
- Alzheimer's disease is the only top ten cause of death in the United States that cannot be prevented, cured or even slowed.
- Eighty-three percent of the help provided to older adults in the United States comes from family members, friends or other unpaid caregivers. Nearly half of all caregivers who provide help to older adults do so for someone with Alzheimer's or another dementia.
- Alzheimer's takes a devastating toll on caregivers. Compared with caregivers of people without dementia, twice as many caregivers of those with dementia indicate substantial emotional, financial and physical difficulties.
- Of the total lifetime cost of caring for someone with dementia, 70 percent is borne by families — either through out-of-pocket health and long-term care expenses or from the value of unpaid care.

The Alzheimer's Association and related organizations maintain up-to-date websites, which are rich in educational material and resources. These notes are included only to provide a broad framework, not definitive information about the subject. This book tells my story as a caregiver and is not intended as a medical resource or manual for caregiving.

Acknowledgments

Shades of Love and Loss is the product of many minds, not just mine. As the author, I am grateful for generous friends and professionals who looked in, shared honest thoughts and contributed countless diverse refinements. I am indebted to each of you for your time, energy, and loving help. Thank you!

Robbee Royce read the first draft of more than three hundred pages and said I had a meaningful book. Her husband had suffered from early-onset Alzheimer's and died before he was 60. She has walked the walk. Robbee's encouragement and skillful editing of many editions midwifed this book. Joanie Forney has been a sister traveler on this journey, not only with the book but also in learning about and managing the dementia-care world. We work as a mini-team to accomplish care-related activities, which softens our on-going grief.

Erica, Rex, Spencer and Karen, my immediate family, and my sister, Judy, have all been pillars of support throughout Dave's journey into dementia. Dave's sister, Nora is part of this group as well. Early in the process, Cousin Carolyn generously offered support through encouragement and sharing her deep experience with dementia caregiving. Karen continues to be instrumental as the boots-on-the ground family member who lives nearby and is on call to help as needed. We each feel the loss of Dave's big presence in our daily lives and do what we can to help each other and Dave.

The support group at Lamorinda Adult Respite Center held and nourished me as I began to comprehend the breadth of impact Dave's illness had on our family and on me. The group offered resources that made immediate and significant difference in my ability to cope.

My friend Melissa Leehan changed her cosmic address while the book was in its earliest form, but for the previous five decades she was my co-conspirator as we faced life's challenges. Her spirit lives throughout these pages.

Jennifer McCord came aboard to assemble and produce the final product. Her professional and personal help has been invaluable in the publishing process. Thank you publicist Mila Fairfax and designer Rudy Ramos as well.

Many thanks to the competent staff and to the residents at Oakmont of Concord for kindness and concern.

Wakyn Ferris, Dave's stepfather, generously included Dave in his will. This inheritance allows us to provide high-level care for Dave and has given me time and space to think and write. I am grateful to him and the Ferris family.

Writing about my family or other people in my life has its challenges. I have altered reality a bit here and there, but not much. I am solely responsible for the content herein.

Nina Krebs
July 17, 2019

For Discussion

The following questions are prompts for conversation in a group or for individuals who are reading this book.

1. Can you relate to the story of SHADES OF LOVE AND LOSS? If so, how so? Directly, on a daily basis, or more generally? Now or sometime in the future?

2. How informed were you about dementia and caregiving before you read the book?

3. Do your perceptions concur or are they different from those of the author?

4. Were there specific passages or stories that were memorable for you? Do they reflect your personal experiences?

5. Did reading the book influence your point of view regarding dementia and caregiving? If so, how is it different now? Can you think of ways you have in common with the author or some that are dissimilar?

6. If you are a caregiver for a partner or someone else with dementia, how have you structured your self-care routine?

7. What support systems are in place for you? Are you able to maintain your routine most of the time? If not, what would help?

8. What are long or short-term consequences for caregiving raised in the book? Are they positive or negative, affirming or difficult?

9. How are you living your story? Do you keep a journal? Attend a support group?

10. Will you think differently or do anything you might not have done after reading this book?

About the Author

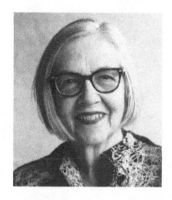

Nina Krebs, a retired psychologist and mother, has been married to Dave Krebs for nearly 50 years. After retirement in 1998, she followed her dreams - as a visual artist, writer and music devotee - until her husband began his journey into the lost land of Alzheimer's. As her world tilted, she intensified her search for meaning. Nina lives in the East Bay area of San Francisco, close to her remarkable family.

CPSIA information can be obtained
at www.ICGtesting.com
Printed in the USA
FSHW021807150819

9 781733 261203